Obesity

Studies in Medical Anthropology

Edited by
Mac Marshall

Advisory Board

William Dressler
Sue E. Estroff
Peter Guarnaccia
Alan Harwood
Craig R. Janes
Sharon Kaufman
Lynn Morgan
Catherine Panter-Brick
Stacy Leigh Pigg
Lorna Rhodes

Obesity

Cultural and Biocultural Perspectives

ALEXANDRA A. BREWIS

RUTGERS UNIVERSITY PRESS

NEW BRUNSWICK, NEW JERSEY, AND LONDON

LIBRARY OF CONGRESS CATALOGING-IN-PUBLICATION DATA

Brewis, Alexandra A., 1965–.
    Obesity: cultural and biocultural perspectives / Alexandra A. Brewis.
       p. cm — (Studies in medical anthropology).
    Includes bibliographical references and index.
    ISBN 978-0-8135-4890-6 (alk. paper)
    1. Obesity—Social aspects. 2. Medical anthropology.   I. Title.
    RC628.B657 2011
    362.196'398—dc22   2010008405

A British Cataloging-in-Publication data for this book is available
from the British Library.

Visit our Web site: http://rutgerspress.rutgers.edu

Manufactured in the United States of America

CONTENTS

FIGURES

TABLES

PREFACE

In this book, I draw on my own and others' research to consider how a cultural or biocultural perspective improves our understanding of obesity as a contemporary phenomenon, using obesity as a revealing lens to explore the current human condition. Obesity is arguably one of the greatest public health challenges we face, rapidly infiltrating almost every aspect of our lives. It shapes who we date, where we work, how much money we make; we are bombarded in the media with messages about the need to be slim and lose weight. In the West, most of us worry about being overweight and work to avoid it, or at least think we should. For many people, obesity is a powerful social symbol of personal failure. It also is understood to represent the very decay of modern life, a sign of how we are damaging ourselves and the world we live in through our collective gluttony and sloth. At the most basic and emotional level, most of us understand that obesity damages us individually and collectively.

Obesity is a topic that seems to resonate with people everywhere. Of all the health-related topics I have worked on over the years—including infertility, family planning, sexually transmitted disease, attention deficit hyperactivity disorder, and depression—obesity is one of the easiest to get people talking about. In my experience, people are usually excited about participating in research in this domain, happy to offer their thoughts and opinions and to be measured. Even in places where obesity is still rare, many are extremely curious about very large bodies. Obesity has a high titillation factor to be sure, but people also attach significant social meanings to those big bodies.

The studies I discuss in this book include a number drawn from my field research over the last two decades in the Pacific Islands, the United States, and Mexico. Mostly by chance, I have run field projects in seven of the twenty fattest countries on earth (see appendix A). If my interest in obesity was seeded at any point early in my career, it was probably during my first trip to Nauru in the late 1980s. A young and very green graduate student at the University of Arizona, heading off for my first long-term fieldwork in the Micronesian nation of Kiribati, I spent several days in the tiny neighboring republic of Nauru awaiting an onward flight. Taking off amid the green sugar cane fields of Fiji, we had been flying across the Pacific Ocean for several hours when a speck of white appeared in the blue—a tiny island, barely a mile across and eight square miles in total. A moonscape stretched across the top of the island, a single road hugged the coastline, and a wide landing strip covered one side.

Nauru, settled by Pacific Islanders for several thousand years, burst upon the world stage in the early 1900s when the expansion of farms in New Zealand and Australia created a high demand for fertilizer, which could be made from the phosphate rock that covered Nauru. By the late 1980s, the phosphate on which the island had been economically dependent for decades was running out. The only unmined rock was beneath the president's home, almost all local food was imported, and the traditional farming and fishing lifestyle had disappeared. Nauru had earned the unfortunate reputation of being the fattest country in the world, with some 80 percent of the population technically obese, based on their estimated body mass index (BMI) of more than $30 \, m/kg^2$ (Coyne 2000).

During my six days waiting for an onward flight, I met a lot of Nauruans, all friendly and mostly very large, and whiled away my time in conversations with them. Many were about food. My field journals show that I wrote extensively, with considerable frustration, about the complete lack of fresh food. That one could find only canned fish on an atoll in the middle of a vast and rich ocean speaks volumes about why people in Nauru are so prone to obesity.

Despite passing through Nauru several times in the next couple of years, my research was in Kiribati, focused on family planning. Kiribati is geographically proximate to Nauru, and the people are genetically, linguistically, and culturally closely related. Many I-Kiribati women were overweight, but despite spending huge amounts of time talking to many people in Kiribati about every possible aspect of their health, I cannot recall obesity being discussed as a health problem even once. Locals saw the big challenge as food shortage, not food excess, in a country with a rapidly expanding population. My conversations about weight were usually with I-Kiribati women, who told me that I was too skinny and would need to fatten up if I ever wanted to attract a husband.

After I completed my dissertation work in Kiribati, I was fortunate to be awarded a postdoctoral fellowship in anthropological demography at Brown University, where I was mentored by biological anthropologist Stephen McGarvey (now the director of Brown's International Health Institute). McGarvey had been running large projects for some years in Samoa and islands in the central Pacific Ocean, focused mainly on issues of cardiovascular disease. Samoans, like the Nauruans, were an unusually overweight population compared to most others globally. They had higher rates of diabetes and hypertension (high blood pressure) and were also in the midst of massive ecological and social changes. McGarvey started working in Samoa as a graduate student at Pennsylvania State University on Paul Baker's human adaptability project (see, e.g., Baker, Hanna, and Baker 1986). Baker's work has helped to shape the way we think about why

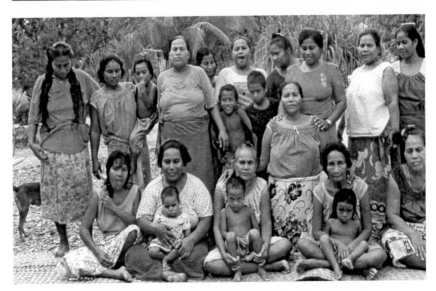

FIGURE PI Women and children in Kiribati in the mid-1990s.
Photo by author.

human bodies vary, understanding growth and development as fundamentally about—and hence reflective of—the process of adapting to local environmental conditions. Baker's research on Samoans, and McGarvey's that followed, had a clear focus on the effects of modernization, which was defined as fundamental changes in technological, social, and economic arrangements that accompany the often rapid transition of small-scale local and regional economies (McGarvey 1992).

Working in Samoa in this context, I started addressing the issue of obesity. My initial foray measured some aspects of Samoan body image cross-culturally, comparing Samoans in less modernized Samoa (then Western Samoa) with the closely related Samoan population in nearby and more developed American Samoa. The Samoans, like the Nauruans, had traditionally placed value on large bodies as high status, and so it seemed an excellent location to consider how views of large bodies might be changing as the country entered the television age and was exposed more frequently to Western ideas about large bodies. I'll talk more about the results of this study in the book, and this opportunity to work (albeit briefly) in the context of those human adaptability studies continues to influence how I conceptualize culture-obesity links.

After leaving Brown, I was hired at the University of Auckland in my native New Zealand, where a large number of Samoans and other Pacific Islanders had migrated in the 1960s in search of work. While living in Auckland for six years, I expanded the Samoan body image project to include Samoans living in

New Zealand. This work included a collaboration with Boyd Swinburn, an endocrinologist then at the University of Auckland School of Medicine, who was interested in community-based research on obesity and diabetes. Coordinating with Swinburn's projects in New Zealand exposed me to an explicit public health approach to obesity, somewhat of an epistemological shock. We were all working on fundamentally the same problem, but I quickly recognized a complete disconnect in how we understood culture. The public health people wanted culture to provide clear, easy, and mainly descriptive answers to why people gained weight or interventions failed. That approach negated everything I found most interesting and powerful about using culture to understand human variation. I suspect my enthusiasm for writing this book in part reflects my desire to move beyond that early-career frustration in trying to reconcile my own intellectual trajectory with what is going on in obesity-related public health.

A fortuitous move to the University of Georgia some fifteen years ago led me to projects that focused on unraveling obesity in different ways. Until then I had viewed myself as a Pacific researcher working on small islands, but in the southeastern United States, I felt it sensible to reorient to something more geographically proximate. My first new project, in collaboration with public health nutritionists in Georgia, focused on understanding the cultural aspects of the very high rate of children's obesity in rural Georgia, which was deeply concerning legislators and public health practitioners. (Georgia was, in fact, in 1999 the first state to legally require insurers to provide coverage for surgical treatment of obesity.) Working with elementary school children, we developed and tested a number of systematic ethnographic techniques for studying cultural ideas about obesity. We started to think about ways to link these techniques more explicitly to questions of biological variation (see, e.g., Brewis and Gartin 2006).

The second project, my main fieldwork at that time, was a large cross-cultural study of behaviors associated with childhood Attention Deficit Hyperactivity Disorder (ADHD). In 2001, I gathered up a field team and headed to Xalapa, the delightful capital of Veracruz state in central eastern Mexico, for six months to collect data on ADHD at a middle-class elementary school. Although Mexico was not identified as having a problem with obesity, the first day we started classroom observations I was thinking about obesity again. Many of the children were overweight, many more than I had seen in Samoa or any of the supposedly "fat" places in which I had worked. It caught me completely by surprise, and I wanted to figure out whether my observations had any explanation.

Anthropometric measures quickly confirmed my initial impressions: over half the boys and a third of the girls were overweight, and some 30 and 20 percent, respectively, were obese. When we interviewed the parents, the majority of those with overweight children did not identify them as having a weight problem. Perhaps because I was pregnant, feeling as fat as could be and hungry all the time, my interest was now truly piqued. My research has focused mostly on obesity, especially in children, ever since.

My most recent move to Arizona State University (ASU) in the large, very western city of Phoenix slightly shifted my research focus again. When I arrived at ASU in 2006, I knew I was here to stay, which meant that I could develop much more complex and ambitious projects that required a longer time frame. I began working with my colleague Seline Szupinski Quiroga, a cultural anthropologist, to identify the health issues that the South Phoenix community expressed as most important. South Phoenix is an area near ASU and south of the downtown, squeezed between the large South Mountain reserve and the interstate highways. The community is currently around 70 percent Latino with some third of its residents born outside the United States (mostly in Mexico), and many households are below the poverty line. Historically, it was the one part of town where minorities could own homes under exclusionary housing covenants. The area has high environmental burdens such as pollution, but also high rates of home ownership and a definite sense of community. These neighborhoods are weathering difficult political and economic storms given the current recession and a massive increase in anti-immigrant policies and enforcement, such as employer sanctions and the aggressive deportation tactics used by the local sheriff's department.

The extended process of interviewing, discussion, and negotiation (sometimes termed community-based research or participatory action research) in South Phoenix identified obesity as a major concern. Starting this project, I had been open minded about what I would end up researching, but I was delighted to have the excuse to dive into the theme of culture and obesity in a much more comprehensive, systematic, and long-term way than I had in the past. Phoenix is an ideal field site because of features such as a sprawling, car-centered built environment and an ecology that discourages physical activity (just try walking or biking anywhere in Phoenix during the summer). We had access to outstanding bioinformatic data, which showed that high rates of diabetes and obesity obtain in most of the low-income areas. All this has facilitated a comprehensive approach to the study of how and why obesity risk is distributed as it is.

If we had gone through the same process with the South Phoenix community a decade ago, I doubt that we would have encountered community-identified concern about obesity. In the nearly twenty years since I first started thinking about the relationship between human biology, culture, and obesity, serious concern with obesity has ballooned in science and medicine, and also in the public consciousness. It is stunning how quickly obesity has gone from being considered an aberration in both popular culture and scientific and public health circles to being perceived as a massive global threat. In the 1980s when I first visited Nauru, the large average size of Nauruans was seen as somewhat anomalous and symptomatic of culturally and biologically unique historical and ecological circumstances. Until that time, most of the limited research into obesity being conducted was focused on a few populations in the Pacific, especially Nauru, as well as on some native American groups, such as the Pima (or Akimel O'odham) and Papago (now known as the Tohono O'odham) of Arizona. These groups were studied because their rates of obesity (and type 2 diabetes) were then so much higher than those of other groups. However, for the most part, obesity was not yet defined as a disease in its own right (Chang and Christakis 2002), and so was mostly discussed as a risk factor for other diseases, such as hypertension and diabetes.

To emphasize how our views of obesity have changed, I remember Steve McGarvey's warning to me sometime around 1992. He told me that obesity was a potentially marginal area for a social scientist to work in, and its explicit study was probably was not the best career move. Even among his anthropologically oriented colleagues at Brown, he explained, talk of fat bodies provoked a nervous titter; obesity was odd, uncomfortable, slightly naughty, and freakish. Now the interest in obesity and obesity funding in academia are proliferating along with the rising size of our bodies. Nauru's early weight gain was, in retrospect, less an aberration than a portent. In an extremely short time, we have made the transition from a species where only a few populations and a few individuals were obese to one in which overweight and obesity have become the norm in many places. The implications of this trend, culturally and biologically profound, provide the impetus for this book.

ACKNOWLEDGMENTS

In writing a book such as this, I am drawing on more than two decades of generous and talented people who have shared ideas, opened doors, endured long interviews, and provided helping hands. In the late 1980s, Bill Stini at the University of Arizona was the first to suggest that looking at bodies and growth was an interesting way to understand human adaptation. In the early 1990s, Steve McGarvey was the first to bring obesity into my line of vision as a scholarly topic, and also very kindly invited me to join his research program in Samoa. John S. Allen introduced me to the benefits of an explicitly evolutionary approach to human behavior and cognition, and Andrea Wiley and Mark Jenike introduced me to the friendly community of nutritional anthropology. Meredith Gartin has worked with me closely over the last ten years on all manner of work related to obesity, first as an undergraduate in my lab and now as a PhD student and full-fledged collaborator. At Arizona State University, Chris Boone opened up to me the parallel universe of human geography and spatial analysis, broadening the ways in which I have been able to think about how culture and biology interact. Seline Szkupinski Quiroga inspires me to pay very close attention to how we can better design our anthropological work on obesity so it actually makes a difference to the communities with which we work. Another intellectually generous colleague, Amber Wutich, has introduced me to the world of social networks. Arizona State is a somewhat unusual institution in its demands that its faculty members work in a trans-disciplinary manner, and its encouragement to focus on basic problems facing society rather than on more parochial disciplinary questions. This creates a supportive and intellectual environment for thinking about a problem like obesity, and I cannot say enough about what a wonderful place the School of Human Evolution and Social Change is for a scholar. I also thank the funding agencies who have supported the research I discuss in this book: the Late Lessons from Early History Presidential Initiative at Arizona State University, the Wenner Gren Foundation for Anthropological Research, the Health Research Council, the Marsden Foundation, the National Science Foundation's cultural and physical anthropology programs, and postdoctoral support through the Andrew W. Mellon Foundation. Laura Sessions, science writer extraordinaire, a long-time collaborator and dear friend, very generously helped with the final revisions.

Writing can also be a very personal act. If I started this book solely as an intellectual exercise, by the end it had become, quite unintentionally, an emotional one. In mid-2008, as the preliminary contract for this book was signed with Rutgers University Press, I was diagnosed with invasive breast cancer. Of all the many new challenges I have had in the last year, the extra abdominal pounds that are one of the side-effects of treatment have—frankly—been the hardest to deal with. If anything, the process of intellectually working through the issues of fat stigma seemed to aggravate my anxieties. My dear friends and family assured me that I was still fabulous even if I was getting fatter. I love them all for trying. At the end of the day, that sort of loving attitude is what helps undo a lot of the fat-focused self-loathing to which many women in our society seem so prone (myself included, apparently).

Finally, I acknowledge my wonderful husband, John Slade, and kids, Olivia and Luke. They allow me to lead a life in which I have the best of circumstances—a warm and fulfilling family life and a fabulously interesting and satisfying career. That comes with some cost to them, and I am incredibly blessed by their generosity.

Obesity

1

Introduction

The Problem of Obesity

The new millennium signaled an important transition for our species. For the first time in human history, in the year 2000 it is estimated that there were more overweight than underweight people globally (Mendez, Monteiro, and Popkin 2005; Worldwatch Institute 2000). According to a recent assessment by the World Health Organization, over a third of people are now overweight or obese. Within two decades, if the current trends continue, the number will be more than two-thirds (Kelly et al. 2008). This is already the case in many industrialized countries, including the United States. In several of the developing nations in the central Pacific, almost the entire adult population is overweight. Even in Africa, a continent usually associated with starvation, obesity is increasing, and the Ugandan Health Institute predicts that obesity-related heart disease will be the leading cause of death in sub-Saharan Africa by 2020 (Berman 2009).

Unlike many other global calamities we are facing (such as climate change), no one predicted the dramatic rise in obesity—in fact, almost no one noticed it until it was well under way. The World Health Organization identified obesity as a major public health problem only in 1997. Johnston and Harkavy (2009, 1) said that neglecting to recognize and address this dramatic rise in obesity in a timely manner was "the greatest public health failure of the past century." The reasons that obesity has increased so dramatically during the last couple of decades have yet to be definitely established (Bray, Nielsen, and Popkin 2004) and the underlying causes remain under contention (Jeffrey and Utter 2003). Research that might help us understand the drivers of the epidemic or even start identifying them is fragmented and weak (ibid.).

However, most scientists attribute the massive increase in obesity during recent decades to changes in environmental conditions, writ broad (French, Story, and Jeffery 2001). The basic reasons we as a species have become fatter during the last three decades are at least generally agreed on: diets emphasizing sugars, fats, and high-calorie liquids; lifestyles tending to the sedentary; increasing and more stable access to low-priced processed foods; and urbanization (Popkin 2009). Bray and Popkin (1998) have demonstrated an association between country-level rates of overweight and fat intake, estimated (albeit crudely) from Food and Agricultural Organization food balance sheets. They argue that the availability of dietary fat (in interaction with more food and more sedentary lifestyles) is a major driver of obesity.

Sobal (2001) agrees that we must look at the Western postindustrial consumer culture and food systems, which now permeate the globe and have made cheap fats and oils easily available. He goes so far as to assert (probably rightly) that the younger members of societies tend to adopt new ideas, such as food preferences or modes of recreation, more quickly and so are at even greater risk than are their parents of suffering from the impact of global processes. Bray, Nielsen, and Popkin (2004) suggest that the ubiquitous high-fructose corn syrup plays a fundamental role in the obesity epidemic, which started at about the same time that high-fructose corn syrup consumption took off (its intake has risen some thousandfold in the United States since 1970). Journalist Michael Pollan has also argued, in *The Omnivore's Dilemma* (2007), that national subsidies of basic crops such as corn and soybeans promote their overuse and create a scenario in which cheap, unhealthy foods become the dietary mainstay, at least in the United States. Another journalist, Greg Critser, in his book *Fat Land* (2003), points to the explosion of poor food and exercise environments— in schools, in front of the television, and in neighborhood fast-food outlets—to explain why such a high percentage of Americans in particular are now overweight. More recently Barry Popkin has made the case, in his deliciously titled book *The World Is Fat* (2009), that another likely culprit is the massive upswing in high-calorie drinks over the last several decades promoted by powerful multinationals. Significant changes in physical activity resulting from the transition from a farming-based to an industrialized economy are also likely involved, but these are much less well documented and understood than the dietary changes (Dufour and Piperata 2008).

In these discussions about the driving forces behind what the World Health Organization has labeled "globesity," several interconnected processes associated with globalization are highlighted, such as mass industrialization, the growth of multinationals, and rapid urbanization. However, these macro-level forces do not affect everyone equally or evenly, even within the same country or city (table 1.1). Understanding how and why the risk of obesity is allocated as it is, and how we can interpret the variation, is a central point of this book. It helps us better understand how obesity can be framed as a social and political— as much as medical—issue. It also helps us think in more sophisticated ways about how we might understand obesity at the community level, which is the

TABLE 1.1

Age-adjusted Distribution of BMI of
U.S. adults, 2006 (in percentages)

	Normal Weight (BMI 18.5–24.9)	Overweight (BMI 25–29)	Obese (BMI ≥30)
Age			
18–44	41.8	33	23.2
45–64	31.4	36.6	30.8
65–74	31.5	39.4	27.5
75 and older	43.4	35.2	18.1
Gender			
Female	43.8	28	25.6
Male	31.9	41.9	25.3
Race/Ethnicity			
Hispanic, Latino	32	39.6	27.4
White	38.2	35.1	25.1
Black	29.5	34.4	34.7
Asian	59.3	27.6	8.3
American Indian; Alaska Native	30	38.1	30.9
Native Hawaiian, other Pacific Islander	29.2	37.6	30.8
Race/Ethnicity by Gender			
Hispanic, Latino: female	36.6	33.1	28.7
Hispanic, Latino: male	27.9	45.8	25.9
White: female	46.2	27.1	23.9
White: male	32	41.9	25.4
Black: female	29.6	28.1	40.6
Black: male	29.4	40.4	28.8
Education			
Less than high school diploma	30.5	38.2	29.7
Bachelor's degree or higher	43.3	35.9	18.8
Income Status			
Poor	36.4	31.6	29.8
Nearly Poor	36.8	33.1	28.5
$75,000+ family income	40.9	35.1	21.9

(continued)

TABLE 1.1

Age-adjusted Distribution of BMI of
U.S. adults, 2006 (in percentages) *(continued)*

	Normal Weight (BMI 18.5–24.9)	Overweight (BMI 25–29)	Obese (BMI ≥30)
Region of Residence			
Northeast	40	34.8	23.6
Midwest	37.2	33.5	27.9
South	36.5	34.9	26.7
West	39.6	36.4	22.1
Place of Residence			
Large Metropolitan Area	39.9	35.4	22.9
Outside Metropolitan Area	33.2	34.4	30.6
All Categories Combined	37.9	34.9	25.5

Source: Centers for Disease Control, http://www.cdc.gov/obesity/data/index.html.

focus of many public health interventions. A clearer picture of who is at risk of obesity helps us better recognize when and where it is most appropriate to focus on the meaning of obesity in social, economic, and cultural terms. Exploring the general patterns of change in obesity risk across space and time also provides a basis for developing theories about why the risk is distributed as it is and how we might unravel the role of culture in its construction and mitigation.

The massive increase in the size of bodies globally during the last two decades, and our reaction to this change, raises a lot of other interesting anthropological questions. Does this massive global rise in obesity substantially alter what we must think of as normal human bodies? Is obesity best conceived as a disease, or an illness, or neither? Is the obesity epidemic really just a huge moral panic best understood in cultural rather than biological terms? What does it mean that minorities and the urban poor are now most at risk for obesity? If most of us are overweight, why does the stigma of being fat persist? If we know how to be slim and want to be slim and have been slim through all our history, why are we getting so fat and unable to shed the excess? Why is obesity such a seemingly intractable bodily state for so many individuals, even when people understand the potential health risks and have all the requisite knowledge on how to lose weight? And, is obesity—viewed from something larger than a purely medical perspective—always a bad thing that needs to be corrected for the sake of the individual, or of society? The answers to these types of questions ultimately tell us something important about what it means to be human—a central concern of my own field of anthropology and the main point of this book. But these answers will also help us better understand obesity as a complex phenomenon, and this has potential quality-of-life implications for many.

Despite the slow start, concern about obesity has proliferated in the last decade or so, focused especially on its health impacts. Obesity has entered the mainstream consciousness and risen to the top of many government and private funding-priority lists. It is identified as "the number one nutritional problem" by the U.S. Department of Agriculture, "a pandemic" (Egger and Swinburn 1997; Prentice 2006), and "globesity" by the World Health Organization. According to the Rand Corporation (Sturm and Wells 2001), the negative health effects of obesity in the United States outweigh the effects of heavy drinking, smoking, or even living in poverty. The U.S. surgeon general has declared obesity more dangerous than terrorism, according to a recent Associated Press wire story. We are told that obesity puts us at elevated risk of hypertension (high blood pressure), osteoarthritis (a degeneration of cartilage and its underlying bone within a joint), dyslipidemia (high cholesterol), type 2 diabetes, coronary heart disease, stroke, gallbladder disease, sleep apnea, respiratory problems (including asthma), and cancers, ultimately leading to more and more complicated and expensive medical treatment, reduced quality of life, and early death.

Phillip James, chair of the International Obesity Task Force, has announced that obesity would soon "overwhelm every medical system in the world," as *USA Today* reported in a September 3, 2006, story headlined "Experts at International Congress on Obesity Warn of Deadly Global Pandemic." Some scientists have expressed concern that life expectancy in the most affluent nations will soon start to decline because of obesity-related disease (Olshansky et al. 2005). Others disagree with this gloomy outlook and point to signs of lifestyle change (Preston 2005) or problems with the scientific evidence supporting this claim (Couzin 2005).

Nonetheless, the reach of obesity is much broader than that of medicine and public health. Widespread obesity is a phenomenon that has managed in a short time to permeate virtually every aspect of our public and private lives (Wadden et al. 2002). If we now spend billions of dollars each year to cover the direct and indirect medical costs of weight-related disease, we lose billions more through decreased work capacity, restricted activity, absenteeism, or lost productivity due to early death (see, e.g., Finkelstein et al. 2003; Wolf 1998; Wolf and Colditz 1998). It is predicted that the figure will soon be in the trillions. Even for developing countries with low obesity rates, scholars such as Barry Popkin (2009) estimate a likely massive increase in obesity during the next few years, with staggering economic costs. For example, he estimates that 9 percent of China's GNP will go toward covering obesity-related economic costs by 2025, even though China has very little obesity at present.

The huge weight-loss industry feeds on concerns about being overweight, and one could label the pursuit of weight loss a national pastime in the United States. Apparently at any single moment, about one quarter of Americans are dieting to lose weight, and more are trying to lose weight by exercising or are thinking about losing weight. North Americans spend some $50 billion annually on products promoted by the ever-burgeoning weight-loss industry, most of which fail to produce the desired outcome. Liposuction, the surgical removal of fat, is now the most common type of cosmetic surgery, and bariatric surgery—stomach reduction—is becoming more common and socially acceptable. Our concerns about weight can be personally consuming, and even as more of us get fat, the stigma against fat people endures. Obesity, "the last socially acceptable form of prejudice" (Sobal and Stunkard 1989), creates enormous social and emotional suffering. The fatter members of our society are statistically more likely to be teased, bullied, and depressed. They are paid less, are less likely to advance in their careers, and have a harder time finding a mate. Our basic sense of self-identity and how we relate to and understand others is increasingly tied to weight.

Given the growing public concern about obesity in recent years, it is no surprise that at the same time we have seen a profligacy of efforts to stall or reverse its rise. These have variously targeted individuals, households or families, schools or other institutions, social networks, communities, neighborhoods, regions, nations, or some combination of these. Yet obesity levels have continued to rise. Slightly more people were—or thought they were—trying to lose weight by diet, exercise, or both in 2000 than a decade earlier (38.5 percent of American adults in 2000 versus 36.6 percent in 1991, according to the Centers for Disease Control's Behavioral Risk Factor Surveillance System); yet over those years U.S. obesity rates rose more than 60 percent and overweight rates went up 16 percent (Mokdad et al. 2003; Tufano and Karras 2005). Studies suggest that public health–based obesity interventions generally fail because they result in little meaningful change in related behaviors (mostly diet and exercise). And despite the billions of additional dollars struggling individuals spend on diet books, frozen dinners, gym memberships, and the exercise equipment gathering dust in a million basements, most of them will regain the weight lost, often plus some extra (Snyder and Hamilton 2002; Tufano and Karras 2005; Weiss et al. 2007).

Traditional media-based public health approaches that promote behavior changes in order to reduce obesity seem to be particularly ineffective. In the early 1990s, the state of California ran a five-year campaign, Five-a-Day for Better Health, that focused on encouraging people to eat more fruits and vegetables. It resulted in no perceptible increase in fruit and vegetable consumption overall, and a significant decrease in fruit and vegetable consumption among some of the most obesity-at-risk groups (for example, Hispanics were down 18 percent; Foerster and Hudes 1989). Similarly, in the late 1990s, a huge three-year public health effort in Europe, Active for Life, focused on increasing the frequency of exercise as part of everyday activities. The result: no measurable change in behavior (Hillsdon et al. 2001).

A reasonably well-developed critique from an anthropological perspective suggests why such public health campaigns seem doomed to failure (see Good 1994; Sobo 2008). The basic conceptual models (such as the health belief model) that dominate public health intervention design focus on the individual as the decision maker and assume that people informed about risks will change their beliefs and hence their behavior (Tufano and Karras 2005). In this way of thinking, "beliefs" is an uncritically applied proxy for "culture" (Good 1994, 39). There are multiple problems with the public health assumption, including a failure to recognize that the decisions we make about our health are not influenced only by individual beliefs (culture). They are also fundamentally structured and constrained by macro-level structural inequalities that in turn reflect and are maintained by social and cultural factors (such as poverty or discrimination).

Another problem here is the common assumption that only other people have culture. For example, obesity researchers might recognize that specific minorities have culture-based ideas that get between them and good health, but completely fail to recognize themselves as operating within and being constrained by a highly culture-bound medical or scientific system. As Sobo (2008, 111) explains: "The belief that only other people have culture continues to thrive in the popular imagination as well as in health services. This is partly because of the invisible, tacit, taken-for-granted nature of culture. Because of this we rarely think about it in reference to ourselves. Unless, that is, it is challenged, for example when faced by a very different dominant culture, such as when we travel. Even then, it is their way that is described as 'cultural,' not our own."

One way that culture influences our thinking about obesity is the core belief that obesity needs to be addressed through personal responsibility, which is actually far more reflective of culture than of the biology of obesity. For example, as Robison et al. (1995, 423) point out: "Conferences continue to include discourses on the failure of traditional weight loss programs, although such lectures would be more appropriately titled 'The failure of fat people to stick to diets.'" Despite the profound effect this culture-laden thinking has on how we understand, organize, and implement obesity prevention and intervention efforts—and likely its critical role in their failures—most in public health do not recognize that this process is occurring.

Further, the notion of culture in public health is often reduced to sets of ideas that can be described, cataloged, and recounted in an organized fashion. As we shall see, some theories of culture support this approach, but in most cases the exercise is at best cursory and in many instances misleading. This approach, which Farmer calls "Anthro Lite" (2005, 15), distracts us from a deeper understanding of the cultural contexts of obesity. For example, focusing on being Latino as a major explanation for the high rates of obesity among Latinos not only is tautological but also stops the search for more comprehensive, and thus ultimately satisfying, explanations. It might be more fruitful to understand how being Latino intersects with structural factors, such as the experience of being a minority in the United States or of having limited access to health care because of immigrant status, income, or location.

Such critical exploration of the failure of traditional public heath interventions is just one of many theoretically sophisticated and potentially useful ways in which we can explore the links between obesity and culture. Culture, it must be recognized, is a basic coalescing idea and organizing principle in anthropology that transects a diverse set of theoretical orientations, and it is accordingly defined and operationalized in a wide range of (not always compatible) ways. I am comfortable with that variety and those contradictions, because looking at the problem of obesity from multiple perspectives tends to enrich our broader understanding. Thus I use the term "culture" in this book in a variety of quite different ways as a means to explore the social contexts of obesity. Culture is an inherently human trait that can both increase our adaptive capacities and act as a stressor in its own right. However, it is also the matrix that shapes the political-economic structures that focus vulnerabilities and reflect the values placed on people because of class, gender, age, or ethnicity. Culture can be understood through such media as stigma, social messaging, and patterned social interaction. Alternatively, it can describe how people perceive and interact with their environments and refer to specific sets of knowledge that people use to make sense of and organize their world. Finally, "culture" can be used in the more prosaic descriptive sense of how and why people interpret and apply various meanings to big/fat bodies. Depending on where you position yourself, obesity might reflect the greatest health challenge of our time, but it might also reflect our remarkable human capacity to accommodate ecological change and adversity, or our equally amazing capacity to institutionalize oppressive social structures that focus risk on the most vulnerable. Obesity might not be "the most serious epidemic ever" but rather a hyperinflated moral panic that is socially rather than physically damaging and best ignored.

We cannot deal with the basic issue here—what it means to be obese—through one approach or perspective or by focusing on one specific aspect of the human condition that deserves a complicated explanation. We too often get stuck in singular theoretical approaches that determine how we think about what is going on in the world. As both a theoretically plural anthropologist and as a pragmatist, all of these ways of thinking about obesity as a human phenomenon—and several others discussed in this book—are potentially correct, proper, and useful; which one is most valuable depends mainly on the question being asked. In the way I approach my science, the most interesting answers often help explain seeming contradictions, or at least accommodate them. It is not that I am merely comfortable with applying sometimes contradictory theoretical views in my research, but also that part of the challenge for me is developing more sophisticated models that can accommodate countervailing forces, feedback loops, and complicated and dynamic processes that make sense even when seen from different viewpoints.

There are good reasons, as I shall explain, to sometimes invoke a specific theory of culture that allows it to be studied in a replicable way, but this is best done within a wider framework that can treat culture as heterogeneous, flexible, and dynamic (e.g., Sobo 2008, 113). Taking such a tack helps us investigate basic questions at the core of my own program of research about how culture becomes literally embodied as obesity. Too often in current anthropology, we do not match our sophisticated theories of culture with a sophisticated capacity to operationalize them. For this reason, I take some time in this book to explain how and why relevant cultural data might be collected in ways that expand our capacity as social scientists to talk about culture in the context of obesity in more systematic and empirical ways. Our texts in anthropology do this far too seldom, and we need to move beyond the methodological mystification that dominates our graduate training.

Rooted in both medical anthropology and human biology, my research fits most comfortably under the moniker "biocultural anthropology," an approach that attempts to understand the iterative and complex interactions between human culture, ecology, biology, and history (including our evolutionary history). For this reason, I pay attention to biological contexts in how I think about the relationships between culture and obesity. Genetics are likely critical to why some people just look at a donut and gain weight and others never seem to gain an ounce regardless of what they eat. Bouchard (2007) reviewed the relevant gene maps for human obesity and concluded that, as of 2005, there were at least twenty-two identified genes governing obesity and energy balance. These could be divided into five main biological propensities: one resembling the thrifty genotype characterized by low metabolic rate, one to do with low or poor appetite suppression, one related to lack of propensity to engage in physical activity, one to do with lipid (fat) metabolism, and one to do with fat storage. From the perspective of human development, we are increasingly aware of how developmental circumstances, especially the role of adverse environments in utero, help to frame obesity risk. The role of human developmental plasticity is well explained in a number of texts, most recently in *The Fetal Matrix* (Gluckman and Hanson 2005). Moreover, some of the potentially useful theories of culture for studying obesity include those that consider our capacity for culture as an evolved set of cognitive skills that adapt us to the demands of our reproductive and social lives (e.g., Swami and Furnham 2008; Tomasello 2008).

Ultimately, though, this book features a purposeful emphasis on the socio-cultural side of the biocultural equation. The transition of our species to massive and widespread fatness has occurred so swiftly and so profoundly that it is necessarily and fundamentally an ecological, social, and cultural rather than an evolutionary phenomenon. There is simply no other way to explain why it has happened so fast and in so many places.

I especially focus on some specific aspects of the culture-obesity connection (especially body image, and to some extent food) at the expense of others (exercise) because my own work has concentrated on these topics. The book is organized to get to what one might think of as the most clearly and classically "cultural" part of an obesity and culture discussion last—the cross-cultural record on how people conceptualize big bodies. This evidence is certainly important in thinking through many of the social aspects of obesity in the modern world, especially its stigmatizing effects. But to really understand the cultural record in relation to obesity in any sort of comprehensive and hence satisfying way, we first must place this variation in the context of both our biologies and ecologies, and consider how and why obesity varies in space and time and across groups. We also need to understand how and why obesity came to be labeled and measured as it is, since this understanding lays the basis for most subsequent discussions about it. This is our starting point in the next chapter.

Many of the approaches introduced in this book are applicable to a wide range of socially focused research on contemporary issues, not just obesity, and in my past and present research collaborations we also apply a number of these methods to such diverse issues as depression, climate change, air and water pollution, antibiotic misuse, and food insecurity. My hope is that this text will be of use to those engaged in community-based health research and intervention who are looking for new or more theoretically expansive and systematic ways to think about, identify, and fix complex contemporary challenges with social bases.

2

Defining Obesity

Most generally, obesity refers to an excess of fat (adipose tissue) storage on the body. Biomedically, obesity in adults is usually understood to mean the level of fat at which health and well-being are adversely affected (Mascie-Taylor and Goto 2007). How obesity is defined technically counts for a lot, because it affects estimates about the condition—whether obesity is becoming more common, and even whether it is a problem at all. Of course, what constitutes an excess of fat—how much fat is too much and when it negatively affects people—is open to considerable debate in both scientific and social terms. Understanding these debates is important to be able to meaningfully interpret data about obesity.

Public agencies globally now monitor obesity because it is seen as a major public health threat. To claim that obesity is increasing globally, or that Nauru has the highest rate of obesity, or that in the United States obesity is associated with some 112,000 excess deaths annually (Flegal, Ogden, and Carroll 2004), or to estimate with any certitude what obesity might be like in the future (Preston 2005), we have to be able to accurately and meaningfully compare and interpret variation in the rates of obesity across space, groups, and time. This requires good referents, agreed-upon standards that allow comparison of one place or time with another on the same terms. For example, in mid-1998, the U.S. government issued new guidelines for the clinical definition of obesity and lowered the definition of overweight from a body mass index (BMI) of 27 m/kg^2 to 25 m/kg^2. With this one action, twenty-nine million more Americans became overweight overnight (NIH and NHLBI 1998). One goal of this chapter is to explain how the common systems for classifying obesity in medicine and public health came to be and how they work.

Another is to explain the basic epidemiological relationships among obesity, disease, and early death to shed light on what is a fairly arbitrary system of defining and classifying obesity as a disease. To cut to the punch line, this chapter not only provides a way to understand how we know what we know about the rise and global spread of obesity risk, but also shows that the scientific and clinical definitions of what an obese body is are somewhat arbitrary.

When thinking about how body fat is estimated and how this translates into the data presented in support of obesity as an epidemic, we need to be careful to talk about age-adjusted prevalence of overweight and obesity, because the overall age structure of populations affects obesity statistics. Generally, people tend to gain weight as they age, with a peak in midlife. Hence we would expect a population with more middle-aged people to have a higher prevalence of obesity than one with more young people, even if every other factor was held constant. Thus, if a population has more forty- to sixty-year-olds and fewer twenty- to thirty-year-olds, the obesity percentages look higher overall. An age adjustment calculates the prevalence of obesity based on how many people are thought to be in an age group (such as from national census counts).

Classifying Obesity by Body Mass Index

Body mass index (BMI) is the most commonly applied measure to estimate adult obesity globally. The idea of BMI was conceived in the mid-1800s by the Belgian statistician, astronomer, and social scientist Adolphe Quetelet, who was searching for a standard measure that could help estimate people's current weight in relation to the ideal weight for their height. BMI has caught on as the most common way to measure levels of body fat in part because it is the easiest. It is based on simple, easily replicated measures of height and weight, it requires no special equipment, and it is highly standardized. BMI is now widely used for medical diagnosis of problematic weight, although it is important to recognize this was not the purpose of its development, and it does not describe individual health risks particularly well (as we shall see). BMI is calculated from an individual's height and weight measurements; it does not directly measure level of body fat. It correlates reasonably well with, but does not exactly overlap, direct measures of body fat.

At the simplest level, BMI is a mathematical indicator of relative weight-for-height of an individual, used as a proxy for the relative amount (usually percentage) of fat on his or her body. It is calculated for adults using a standard formula (table 2.1) that divides weight by height squared. A shortcut is to calculate BMI (say, for a person who is 5′ 5″ tall and weighs 180 pounds) by multiplying weight in pounds by 703 (180 × 703 = 126,540) and square height in inches (65 × 65 = 4225), then divide the first result by the second (126,540 ÷ 4,225 = BMI of 29.9). You can also use a chart (see appendix B) to estimate your classification based on height and weight.

TABLE 2.1

Formulas for Calculating BMI and Body Fat Percentage

To calculate BMI in kilograms and meters (divide height in centimeters by 100 to obtain height in meters): BMI = weight (kg) ÷ [height (m)]^2

Example: If weight = 68 kg and height = 165 cm (1.65 m),
then BMI = 68 ÷ (1.65)^2 = 24.98

To calculate BMI in pounds and inches: BMI = weight (lb) / [height (in)]^2 × 703

Example: if weight = 150 lbs and height = 5′ 5″ (65″),
then BMI = [150 ÷ (65)^2] × 703 = 24.96

To convert BMI to a body fat percentage (percentage of total weight taken up as fat): *Body fat percent* = 1.2 * BMI + 0.23 * *age* − 5.4 − 10.8 * *gender*, where gender is 0 if female and 1 if male. This takes into account that body fat percentage is about 10% greater in women than in men at the same BMI, and that percentage of body fat tends to go up with age even if BMI does not.

The most widely applied and accepted system for translating BMI measures to categories of overweight and obesity is the shared classificatory system published in the late 1990s by the National Institutes of Health and World Health Organization (e.g., WHO 1998). The system is based on large-scale epidemiological studies demonstrating a relationship between levels of BMI and elevated premature death, as considered and interpreted by an unpaid expert panel primarily of scientists. People are classified into one of four basic categories: underweight, normal, overweight, or obese (see table 2.2). Overweight status is assigned to anyone with a body mass index between 25 and 29.9, because this is the size at which there was an increased risk of mortality within studied populations. Obese status is applied to those with a BMI at or above 30, because the risk of mortality increases further above this size. A BMI between 18.5 and 25 is considered normal weight, and under 18.5 is classed as underweight. Being underweight is considered less than ideal because it too is associated in a very general way with increased mortality risk.

Using these cutoff points to define overweight and obesity (i.e., BMI of 25 and 30 respectively) is a useful heuristic because it is simple and easy to estimate. The selection of 25 and 30 as cutoff points is based in part on their simply being round numbers (Cole et al. 2000). However, there are three other basic and less arbitrary rationales used to derive these cutoff points from existing datasets to relate weight to elevated health: risk-based, prescriptive, and statistical (see Pelletier 2006 for a more extensive discussion). The risk-based approach is based on estimates of the level of adiposity at which health or life span is adversely affected. The prescriptive approach is based on an idea of

TABLE 2.2

**Common Weight Classifications, Associated BMIs, and
Assumed Associations with Early Mortality Risk**

Weight Classification	BMI	Early Mortality Risk Level
Underweight	Below 18.5	Increased
Normal weight	18.5–24.9	Average
Overweight or pre-obese	25–29.9	Increased
Obesity (class I)	30–34.9	High
Obesity (class II)	35–39.9	Very high
Extreme obesity (class III)	40 or above	Extremely high

Source: From National Institutes of Health and National Heart,
Lung, and Blood Institute 1998.

how we should grow rather than how we actually do grow. The statistical approach determines the distribution of adiposity in a population and defines overweight and obesity in relation to a specified population mean. Risk-based and prescriptive approaches both demand significant epidemiological data on related risks. Generally, approaches to adult obesity classification are risk based, while a mix of all three approaches is used for classifying childhood overweight and obesity. A significant technical challenge underlying all these approaches is that they necessitate, by implication, the recognition that there are two groups of people within any population sample: those who are healthy (i.e., normal weight), and those who are not (i.e., overweight, obese, or underweight).

The historical rationale underlying the selection of 30 as a BMI cutoff point for adult obesity relies on a risk-based model: a BMI of 30 is the level at which adiposity becomes associated with significantly elevated disease risk (particularly, in fact, premature mortality). This cutoff point is essentially based on eyeballing the curve flexion to estimate where there is a sense of increasing mortality related to increased size (Garrow and Webster 1985; Mascie-Taylor and Goto 2007; see figure 2.1 for an example). Given these are based on pooled data, there are some real problems with using these types of information to predict *individual* disease risk.

One of the main concerns with using BMI to assess obesity in individuals is that the weight measures do not distinguish between weight comprised of fat and that comprised of muscle, bone, cartilage, and water weight, especially in overweight or mildly obese individuals (Romero-Corral et al. 2006). In other words, BMI measures do not distinguish big bodies from fat ones, and so are particularly problematic when used to define individuals (versus populations) as obese (and at risk). Thus while BMI might be a reasonable estimator of obesity levels in and across populations, it is limited in its ability to accurately estimate whether an individual has excess fat.

Muscle is much denser and weighs more than fat, and so very muscular, lean people such as many athletes can have very high BMIs. People who qualify as obese based on their BMI include many Olympic medal winners and Governor Arnold Schwarzenegger at his physical peak. At 5′ 11″ and 187 pounds, actor Matt Damon is classified "overweight" with a BMI of 26, as is 6′ 2″, 210-pound actor Will Smith, who clocks in with a BMI of 27. Actor George Clooney, at 5′ 11″ and 211 pounds, is almost obese with a BMI of 29. These examples illustrate that one problem in reading both individual and population assessments of obesity based on BMI is that people are assigned to overweight and obese categories without any consideration of their normal exercise patterns. BMI measures thus capture "high adiposity" best when applied to those who are relatively sedentary (WHO 1995).

Using BMI to define obesity is additionally problematic because the measures do not consider how gender, age, and population history affect body mass. At the same BMI, women in general have more body fat than men have, and older people, on average, tend to have more body fat than do those who are younger. Furthermore, risk of obesity rises with age, although it peaks in the forty- to sixty-year-old window. The most recent National Health and Nutrition Examination Survey analyses show that being forty to eighty years of age puts an individual at about 2.5 times (female) or 3 times (male) the risk of being overweight or obese compared to someone who is between twenty and forty years of age. But for those over eighty years of age, especially women, the risk is not statistically different from that of twenty- to thirty-nine-year-olds (Ogden et al. 2006, table 6).

Population-level variation in the relationship between actual body fat levels and BMI is widely recognized. Deurenberg, Yap, and van Staveren (1998) conducted a meta-analysis (a study pooling data from similar studies) that tested whether the relationship between BMI and percentage body fat measured by direct means was the same across diverse populations. In fact, they found some significant differences. For example, in a comparison of European-derived populations with Polynesians of the same directly measured percentage of body fat, at the same age and of the same gender, the calculated Polynesian BMIs based just on height and weight were 4.5 kg/m² lower than that of European-ancestry samples. African American BMIs were 1.3 kg/m² higher and Indonesian BMIs 3.2 kg/m² lower than European BMIs. Thus, the standard BMI formula, compared to direct and accurate measures of body fat, tends to underestimate the percentage body fat of Asians, but to overestimate that of Polynesians (Swinburn, Amosa, and Bell 1999).

Deurenberg, Yap, and van Staveren (1998) conclude, and many others agree, that this finding has important public health implications for BMI levels used to define overweight and obesity. For example, they suggest that the cutoff defining Polynesians as obese should be above the standard 30 kg/m², but for Indonesians it could appropriately be as low as 27 kg/m². Lowering the cutoff point for Singapore from 30 to 27 kg/m² would increase the percentage of obese in that country from 6 percent to 16 percent (Deurenberg-Yap 2000). The World Health Organization, the International Association for the Study of Obesity, and the International Obesity Task Force have all recommended that for Asian populations in particular, the cutoff for obese class I should now be set at a BMI of 25, with that for overweight at a BMI of 23 (e.g., WHO 2004), although this distinction is rarely applied in scientific studies. There is also some evidence that Asian Americans reach the same risk of diabetes at a significantly lower BMI than other groups, meaning that their overall lower BMI does not necessarily mean they are at lower health risk (McNeely and Boyko 2004). However, a couple of more recent studies in Asian populations have found that the relationship between a given level of BMI and mortality risk was not significantly different from that of other populations (Gu et al. 2006 for China; Jee et al. 2006 for Korea).

Differences in body proportions also affect the relationship between BMI and body fat (Norgan 1994). A person with a stocky build tends to have more connective tissue and muscle mass than does a slender person of the same height. Thus, the slender person has more body fat at the same BMI. Relative leg length, usually measured as sitting height (the distance from top of the head to the seat surface when sitting upright), figures into this calculation, because a leg length shorter in relation to overall body height results in a higher BMI, even if you hold percentage body fat constant (Bogin and Beydoun 2007; Norgan and Jones 1995). In other words, a person with long legs tends to have a lower BMI than someone with the same degree of adiposity and of the same height who has shorter legs and hence a comparatively longer trunk.

Just being taller also makes a difference in BMI. Mathematically, the reason tall people have lower relative BMIs is that for a body height, shape, and density, BMI is proportional to weight. However, for a body fixed on weight, shape, and density, BMI is inversely proportional to the square of the height. It should be noted, though, that short people are not just scaled-down versions of tall people, but tend to have wider frames proportionate to height.

These differences can have important implications for interpreting BMI across populations as well as within them, because groups with diverse population histories can have quite different average or modal body shapes (Eveleth and Tanner 1976). Allen's Rule describes a biogeographic pattern in which people derived from populations adapted to cold climates (such as Inuit) tend to have shorter legs and arms relative to their overall height, and those from warm climates (such as the Sudan) tend to have relatively long arms and legs. Thus one would expect Alaskan natives and East African tribespeople with the same percentage body fat to have higher and lower BMI measures respectively.

Consider the case of people native to Tonga, an island kingdom next to Samoa in the south-central Pacific Ocean. Compared to Australians, Tongans have shorter legs relative to trunk length and significantly lower percentage of fat levels at the same BMI. For example, at a BMI of 30, a Tongan woman has on average 37 percent body fat, compared to 43.5 percent in a similarly aged Australian woman with the same BMI (Craig et al. 1999). Tongan men at BMI 30 have 24 percent body fat, versus 34 percent in Australians. To match the percentage body fat of someone with a BMI of 30 in Australia, a Tongan would need to have a BMI of just over 35.

This variation has implications for understanding the very high levels of obesity reported among Pacific Islanders based on their high average BMIs. In a sample of Samoan adults in our 1994 body image study (Brewis et al. 1998), the BMI of participants ranged from 19 to almost 50. Taking the standard BMI cutoff point of 30, the prevalence of obesity (percentage of the sample who are obese) is 50.6 percent. If we adjust the cutoff point for obesity upward by 4.5 to a BMI of 34.5, then the prevalence of obesity halves to 24.7 percent. These data suggest that Pacific Islanders may not be the fattest populations globally but rather have the highest mean body masses. In addition, Polynesians tend to have larger skeletal frames than other populations have, which would increase BMI values relative to percentage body fat (see, e.g., Craig et al. 2001).

Alternative Methods for Estimating Body Fat

Different methods of estimating body fat may be useful depending on the purpose for collecting the measures (see table 2.3). BMI is a useful, easy-to-apply method, but it has limitations, including that it does not directly measure fat levels in the body. A number of other methods can more directly assess the relative amount of adipose tissue on our bodies, or our body composition, and these are often more appropriate for scientific research or clinical practice because they tend to be more accurate. However, they also often require additional equipment and training.

The most common method for measuring body fat percentage is to use calipers to measure the thickness of subcutaneous fat in different places on the body. This method captures the percentage of fat in the body, as about half our fat sits right below the skin, although the distribution varies based on factors such as gender, age, and ethnicity (Malina 1996). The most commonly used skin folds include those above the triceps and biceps on the upper arm, one in the subscapular area on the back, and the supra-iliac skin fold at the top of the pubis on the stomach area. Among biocultural anthropologists, nutritional

TABLE 2.3

Relative Utility of Methods for Measuring Body Fat

Method	Utility of Measurement		
	For total body fat	*For regional fat distribution*	*In field-based studies*
Anthropometry			
Body mass index (BMI)	Moderate	Very low	Very high
Waist and hip measures	Low	High	Very high
Skinfolds	Moderate	Moderate	High
Bioelectrical impedance analysis (BIA)	Moderate	Very low	High
Dual X-ray absorptiometry (DXA)	Very high	Very low	Low
Magnetic resonance imaging (MRI)	High	Very high	Low
Computed tomography (CT)	Moderate	Very high	Low
Body Volume 3D Scanning	High	Very High	Low

Source: Adapted from Snijder et al. 2006, table 1.

anthropologists, and human biologists who do fieldwork, taking skin-fold thickness measures is the agreed standard to assess nutritional status, including obesity and the one I have used most often in my projects. The main advantage of this technique is that one can capture total body fat and distribution fairly well under even difficult field conditions; the equipment is easy to carry, the method is minimally invasive for participants, and training in the technique is reasonably simple. However, skin folds can be difficult to measure in very large people because it is tricky to grasp the fat properly with the calipers.

For work in a clinical or laboratory setting, a number of other methods can be used. Bioelectrical impedance analysis measures the resistance of electrical flow through the body to estimate body fat, because electricity flows more easily through fat than through muscle. Hydrostatic weighing, in which individuals are sunk into a large tank of water to see how well they float (fat floats, muscle sinks), is an especially accurate way to assess percentage of body fat, although because of the obvious impracticalities the technique is seldom used. Also often impractical is air weighing, which assesses body composition via measure of body density and requires a special sealed chamber. Another increasingly applied and particularly accurate laboratory and medical scanning technique for measuring fat mass and body fat percentage, as well as for assessing variation in fat levels across different regions of the body, is dual X-ray absorptiometry (Kiebzak et al. 2000). The most accurate ways to measure body composition are magnetic resonance imaging (MRI) and computed tomography (CT), but both are unwieldy and expensive.

New technologies being developed include body mass volume measures (Body Volume Index, or BVI) that use 3D scanning to examine both volume and weight distribution, assessing where fat is deposited on the body rather than total weight or total fat content. A large international study, the Body Benchmark Study, was begun in 2007 to establish the potential value and feasibility of testing BVI in health care settings. The cumbersome equipment required means BVI will probably never be a useful method for field-based studies.

Categorizing Childhood Overweight and Obesity

The notions of overweight and obesity are even more complicated for children than for adults and are assessed somewhat differently. Children's bodies undergo many changes during growth, and the health consequences of adiposity in childhood are not at all obvious. What constitutes an unhealthy level of fat varies quite markedly with age and by gender throughout childhood and adolescence. Thus, the presence of overweight and obesity in children and adolescents is often assessed using the same BMI formulas used for adults, but the results are interpreted and used somewhat differently.

In children under eighteen, by-age measures are used to classify overweight and obesity by comparison to standardized growth charts. This method recognizes that what constitutes a normal or healthy weight changes month to month in childhood, given that children are growing. The growth charts allow one to estimate overweight based on a child's size at any age compared to a reference sample. For example, a fifteen-year-old boy with a BMI of 23 would be classified as normal weight because he is close to the expected median for a boy that age, whereas a ten-year-old with the same BMI would be classified as obese because his body mass is much higher than the reference median. The reference curves are also distinguished by gender because there are significant differences between girls and boys in their normal patterns of growth, and in the sequence and patterning of fat deposition as children mature through adolescence. For example, girls typically gain pubertal fat earlier than boys do. The references are used to calculate a percentile for a child's individual measures that corresponds to where that child sits within a larger population.

The most commonly used charts for children in the United States were developed on the basis of children's (ages two to twenty years) height and weight data collected since the early 1960s in the large-scale National Health and Nutrition Examination Survey (NHANES). The NHANES collects directly measured height, weight, skin fold, and some other measures such as waist circumference (see NHANES 2007). Newer charts released by the Centers for Disease Control (CDC) based on U.S. data excluded very low birth weight, premature infants (born at less than 1500 grams) and are more representative of the country's ethnic diversity and current breastfeeding practices (Ryan, Roche, and Kuczmarski 1999). These charts reflect a change in thinking about what normal growth is for children, because breast-fed children tend to weigh less and gain weight more slowly early in life.

In 1993, the World Health Organization noted that the U.S.-based charts did not make much sense for non-U.S. populations, whose growth trajectories can be very different. WHO subsequently developed the Multicentre Growth Reference Study, a community-based, multicountry project undertaken to improve the growth reference standards for infants and young children across a wide variety of populations. Rather than devise an average of how all children were growing, the project took pains to identify an *ideal* of child growth, that is, to identify heights, weights, and thus BMIs by age for a sample of children growing under what could be considered ideal circumstances. These circumstances included being breast-fed, not suffering from poor diet or infection, getting adequate health care, and not having a mother who smoked. The sample of 8,440 children was drawn from six countries: Brazil, Ghana, India, Norway, Oman, and the United States. The new curves, introduced in 2007, tend to result in higher estimates of the prevalence of overweight and obesity compared to the CDC reference curves.

The U.S.-based child growth reference approach uses a statistical model to define child obesity, identifying how an individual's measurements relate to those of the sample population and statistically determining where the individual sits relative to everyone else. Currently, CDC and WHO practice is to define as overweight children above the 85th percentile for BMI by age and as obese those at the 95th percentile or above. Unlike the adult estimators, these cutoff points are not derived from any particular evidence that children at this level of adiposity face additional health risk. Instead, by being at or above the 95th percentile, the child in question simply has a higher BMI than 95 percent of children that are the same gender and age.

The charts most commonly used in doctors' offices to track children's height and weight, originally issued by the National Center for Health Statistics (NCHS), also use the 85th and 95th percentiles as cutoff points to define overweight and obesity respectively in children. The NCHS growth curves are based on data collected starting in the 1960s when the average child weighed much less than the average child today. Clearly, if the references continue to be updated as the average size of children goes up, then the number of children

TABLE 2.4

**Comparison of U.S. and U.K. Measures of
Childhood Overweight and Obesity**

CDC BMI category	UK Weight Status Category	CDC BMI-for-Age Percentile	CDC BMI-for-Age z-score
Underweight (<18.5 BMI)	Underweight	< 5th	> 2 SD below
Healthy or normal weight (18.5–24.9 BMI)	Healthy or normal weight	5th to < 85th	< 1 SD below or < 1 SD above
Overweight (25–29.9 BMI)	"At-risk for overweight"	85th to < 95th	> 1 SD above[a]
Obese (>=30 BMI)	Overweight	≥ 95th percentile	> 2 SD above[b]

Note: SD = standard deviation.
[a] Equivalent to BMI of 25 at age 19
[b] Equivalent to BMI of 30 at age 19

above the 85th percentile, and thus defined as overweight, will be revised sharply downward.

The way childhood overweight and obesity are defined varies markedly across countries, even between the United States and United Kingdom, as shown in table 2.4. This variation further complicates discussions of global childhood obesity, because public health authorities using the same methods may apply different cutoff points. For example, in France the accepted limit for childhood overweight is the 90th percentile, and for obesity the 97th percentile (Rolland-Cachera et al. 1991).

Why do we use the 85th, 90th, 95th, and 97th percentiles, apart from convention? Are adult BMI standards of any use for measurement in children if they are based on health or mortality effects that are absent, or at least very different, in childhood (Cole et al. 2000)? We currently have no satisfying answer to either question. As a result, Cole and colleagues (2000) developed a useful comparative reference for estimating overweight and obesity in childhood at various ages that can compare to the adult cutoff points of 25 and 30 (see appendix B, table 2). The estimator is useful because it moves away from the arbitrary use of specific percentiles for estimating obesity in children, which fail to account for the substantial age-related change of means of body mass index in childhood; for example, expected growth curves rise rapidly for most children between birth and one year of age. The estimator also makes the cutoff points for children more comparable to those for adults and makes the measures applicable to use as a reference for ideal or expected growth patterns in childhood in a wider range of populations, not just data from the United States.

Does Obese Equal Unhealthy?

In biomedicine, a widely understood and often expressed theory holds that excess fat in later adulthood causes major and profound disease. A long laundry list of the disease conditions that reputedly result from excess fat and therefore shorten the lifespan of overweight and obese individuals includes hypertension (elevated blood pressure), dyslipidemia (for example, high LDL cholesterol, low HDL cholesterol, or high levels of triglycerides), type 2 diabetes, coronary heart disease, congestive heart failure, stroke, gallbladder disease, osteoarthritis, sleep apnea, respiratory problems, and some cancers (especially endometrial, postmenopausal breast, gallbladder, and colon). Other conditions associated with reduced functioning in overweight and obese people include gallstones, polycystic ovarian syndrome, pregnancy complications (such as gestational diabetes), hirsutism (excess hair), stress incontinence, and depression.

Sometimes the causal relationship between obesity and health abnormalities can be difficult to decipher. For example, consider the metabolic syndrome, which is a common medical diagnosis for a cluster of health abnormalities, primarily including insulin resistance and abdominal fat, as well as hypertension, atherogenic dyslipidemia (lipid abnormalities), prothrombotic state (predisposal to clots within a blood vessel), and proinflammatory state (slow healing). Approximately 22 percent (47 million) of the U.S. adult population is estimated to have this syndrome (Ford et al. 2002). However, medical practitioners argue over whether the syndrome is a *result* of obesity or a corollary of a much more profound metabolic disturbance that *leads* to obesity and a host of related problems. There is also argument about whether metabolic syndrome is more than the sum of these parts or a set of cardiovascular disease risk factors that tend to cluster together (Kahn 2008).

While exact cause and effect remain undemonstrated for many conditions as a function of obesity, there is good evidence that, following weight loss, most or all of these conditions tend to diminish or reverse (NIH and NHLBI 1998). So, how definitive are the epidemiological data linking various levels of disease or mortality to variation in BMI or other estimators of adiposity? There is no doubt that being very obese has some substantial negative health consequences. Although the results vary depending on the population studied and the methods applied, some convincing scientific evidence points to a relationship between level of adiposity and increased risk of dying at various ages (Stevens,

McClain, and Truesdale 2006). However, the relationship is not straightforward. In particular, the pattern is nonlinear, meaning that it is not simply a function of health getting worse with each percentage point of fat added.

Furthermore, some studies have failed to find a link between obesity and increased mortality. In a meta-analysis of forty studies totaling some 250,000 participants, Romero-Corral et al. (2006) found no real and consistent evidence linking overweight and obese categories based on BMI to worse health and survival compared to normal weight categories. In fact, the relative risk of mortality was lowest in those classified as overweight and obese compared to all other groups, and highest in those who were underweight. (It is interesting to consider why the cultural concern regarding the mortality risk associated with being underweight is less than for the overweight, if the health and survival costs appear high for both categories.) Even severe obesity failed to make a difference in mortality risk. Considering only deaths caused by coronary artery disease, the severely obese were at greater risk, but the obese and overweight had no greater chance of dying than those at normal sizes.

The failure to find consistent evidence for increased mortality in overweight and mildly obese individuals may be due partly to differences in the accuracy of measurements used to define overweight and obesity categories (Romero-Corral et al. 2008). A recent study found that obesity defined by BMI measures was much lower (19.1 percent of men and 24.7 percent of women) than obesity identified using the more direct method of bioelectrical impedance analysis (43.9 percent of men and 52.3 percent of women). The difference in accuracy was especially problematic at moderate BMI levels of 25–29.9 (the overweight category). Therefore, the way obesity is categorized using BMI may simply fail to capture many of those at risk because of excess fat. Physical activity may also have a major .ugating influence on whether fat is associated with increased mortality and morbidity, because those who exercise may be at reduced risk once body fat is controlled for (Blair and Brodney 1999; Katzmarzyk, Janssen, and Ardern 2003; cf. Hu et al. 2004; Orsini et al. 2008).

The relationship between obesity and health is even less clear in children. There is a tracking effect between being overweight as a child and overweight as an adult, and this certainly seems to elevate the risk of such conditions as diabetes and cardiovascular disease in later life (Dietz 1998). A recent and important review of published studies concluded, however, that there is little evidence to suggest that childhood obesity or overweight in and of itself leads to an elevated risk of adult disease or elevated risk of dying sooner (Lloyd, Langley-Evans, and McMullen 2009). The reviewers found that once adult BMI was controlled for, studies showed cumulatively that cardiovascular risk in adulthood is best explained by the tracking of higher BMI from childhood into adulthood. They also concluded that the studies showed that the risk of high blood pressure in adults is in fact greatest in those who were skinniest in childhood but became

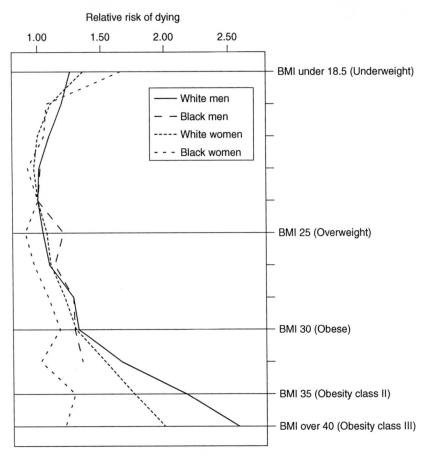

FIGURE 2.1 Relative risk of dying by body mass index (BMI) categories. Data selected from a prospective study of more than one million adults in the United States includes only nonsmokers (Calle et al. 1999). The relative risk of dying at each level of BMI category is by comparison with those in the 23.5–24.9 (upper normal weight) category.

overweight as adults. This does not mean that interventions to reduce child-hood overweight and obesity are misguided, since they should help prevent tracking into adulthood, but it does challenge much of the standard medical thinking that childhood obesity is extremely concerning on its own as a con-tributor to later-life disease.

It is also quite possible to have reasonably high levels of body fat, even to be technically obese, and be metabolically healthy. Although obesity is often asso-ciated with cardiovascular disease risk, insulin resistance, and other metabolic disorders, there is a distinct set of people defined as obese on the basis of their weight who are "metabolically normal" based on accepted cutoff points for insulin sensitivity, a standard metabolic marker of diabetes risk (8 mg/min * kg

LBM [lean body mass]; Brochu et al. 2001). A 2008 study using NHANES 1999–2004 data for a large sample of U.S. adults compared indicators of metabolic health (blood pressure, triglycerides, blood sugar, and "good" cholesterol) among adults who were defined by their BMI as obese, overweight, or normal (Wildman et al. 2008). The study found that half of overweight adults and a third of obese adults were metabolically healthy, and a quarter of the normal weight adults had readings considered unhealthy. In other words, one can have a normal weight but have the health profile normally associated with someone larger, or one can be obese but have a healthy biomarker profile. What appeared to improve a person's health profile even at larger sizes was having less abdominal fat (smaller waist diameter), exercising more, and being younger. A recent Mayo Clinic study reports that of a sample of just over two thousand individuals classified normal weight based on their BMI, more than half had blood chemistry that suggested they were obese, such as high cholesterol, high leptin, and high rates of the metabolic syndrome (Romero-Corral et al. 2008).

This study and others show that, in terms of risk assessment, the emphasis on overweight and obesity based on BMI means that quite a number of people at risk for cardiovascular disease probably fail to see themselves as being so. As studies increase in number and size, we are gaining a better appreciation of how obesity and disease are linked, and the relationship is neither linear nor simple. Certainly, having a BMI of 30 transfers very little, if any, additional risk over someone with a BMI of 28 or 29, but the disease profile of someone with a BMI of 23 usually (but not always) looks very different than that of someone with a BMI of 43. Importantly, there are also results showing a high prevalence of that metabolic syndrome in a number of well-studied populations in Asia, where obesity is relatively rare, albeit increasing (e.g., Hsieh and Muto 2006).

Fat distribution across different areas of the body, rather than overall levels of fat, may also be extremely important for defining physical health risks. As noted, BMI-based measurements do not capture fat distribution well. For this reason, waist diameter is often used as a simple additional anthropometric assessment of potential disease risk. High abdominal fat content (including visceral and, to a lesser extent, subcutaneous abdominal fat) is highly correlated with a worse metabolic profile and more obesity-related health complications (table 2.5). The so-called android (male) pattern of fat deposition around the abdomen (such as a beer belly) in particular appears to lead to worse comparative health outcomes than the gynecoid (female) pattern of obesity that is focused in the hips and backside.

The generally applied cutoff points for cardiovascular risk in clinical settings are a waist circumference greater than 94 centimeters (37 inches) in men and greater than 80 centimeters (31.5 inches) in women and a waist-to-hip ratio greater than 0.95 in men and greater than 0.80 in women. Very high risk based on these measures is generally accepted to be a waist circumference of 102 cm

TABLE 2.5

Comorbidity Risk Calculated by BMI and Waist Circumference

	Comorbidity Risk	
BMI	*Waist circumference < 90 cm (men); < 80 cm (women)*	*Waist circumference > 90 cm (men); > 80 cm (women)*
Below 18.5	Low (but not negligible)	Average
18.5 to 24.9	Average	Increased
25–29.9	Increased	Moderate
≥ 30	Moderate	Severe

Source: Adapted from WHO 2000, table 2.2.

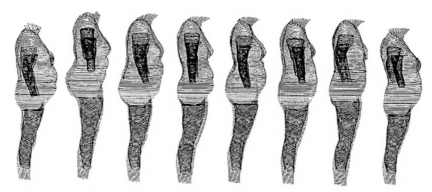

FIGURE 2.2 The possible distribution of fat deposits on a woman with a body mass index of 30. Figures with more central, abdominal fat incur a higher relative disease risk, even with the same BMI as other figures.

(40 inches) in men and 88 cm (35 inches) in women. BMI, of course, does not discriminate in this way, which is why clinical and research practice increasingly combines BMI with a waist measurement to assess disease risk. This method perhaps is most important for examining individuals who are overweight or slightly obese. Figure 2.2 shows the shape of eight different women who all have a BMI of 30 but quite different patterns of fat distribution. An approach that takes into account waist circumference would suggest that the women at both ends of the figure, who carry proportionately more of their

weight abdominally, are most at risk for hypertension, stroke, and heart disease, as well as glucose intolerance and other metabolic diseases.

There is also growing thought that waist-to-height ratio might be a better single measure of how much fat is too much. A 2008 study by Gelber and colleagues examined the relationship of four measures of adiposity—BMI, waist circumference, waist-to-hip ratio, and waist-to-height ratio—and risk of cardiovascular disease (CVD) in two very large U.S. studies. They found that waist-to-height ratios had the strongest relationship to CVD risk, but also notably that all the measures were linearly associated with increased risk of CVD; as fat measures went up so did apparent health risks.

The link between health outcomes and adiposity may also in part be explained by a person's energy balance rather than simply by level of fat (Stevens, McClain, and Truesdale 2006), or by confounding factors such as smoking that account for higher mortality at lower BMIs. A recent study of Seventh Day Adventist men (who neither drink nor smoke) showed the lowest risk of mortality at BMI of less than 20 (Lindsted, Tonstad, and Kuzma 1991). In contrast, a study using data from the NHANES surveys concluded that persons overweight but not obese (BMI between 25 and 30) were at lower risk of mortality than were underweight individuals, especially after age seventy (Flegal, Ogden, and Carroll 2004). Compared to being normal weight, being overweight was not more risky, but being either obese or underweight had negative health consequences. Thus, based on what we know at present about risk of premature death and body size, normal weight does not necessarily equal a healthy weight, and "normal weight obesity" is starting to enter medical parlance. Viewed another way, it is quite possible to be obese even if one is normal weight, if obesity is defined as having very high body fat and the associated clinical disease markers.

However, another key aspect of the health impact of obesity is often overlooked, despite its being one of the most consistently observed health correlates of being very overweight, at least in the industrialized West: growing evidence suggests that obesity may lead to higher rates of depression and other mood disorders. In the National Comorbidity Survey replication, which collected self-reports of height and weight and depression symptoms from nearly ten thousand (educated, mostly white) Americans, obese men and women (BMI > 30) had a 20 to 50 percent higher prevalence of mood and anxiety disorders than normal weight individuals (Simon et al. 2006).

The causal pathways that link obesity to depression are not well understood and probably iterative; there is evidence that depression can precipitate obesity, just as obesity can cause depression. Moreover, depression appears to make weight loss much more difficult, and weight loss is often observed to relieve depression. Combining data from sixteen longitudinal studies, Blaine (2008) found that depressed adolescents were more than 2.5 times more likely to become obese over time compared to other adolescents. Atlantis and Baker

(2008) reviewed the epidemiological evidence suggesting that obesity led to depression and found a positive association but not enough evidence for direct causation because of the lack of longitudinal data. If there are clear causal links between obesity and depression, they could be mediated by several underlying mechanisms: both depression and anxiety are related at some level to dysregulation of stress systems and appear to have some shared relationships to a number of neuropeptidergic and neurotransmitter systems involving chemicals that help to regulate mood and body weight (Bornstein et al. 2006).

The Medicalization of Obesity

The bigger question, then, is whether classifying obesity using BMI or percentage of body fat is meaningful. Paul Campos, a law professor at the University of Colorado, has been particularly critical of the focus on BMI as the basis for public discussions about obesity as ill health (Campos 2004; Campos et al. 2006). To him, the problem is not just classificatory or semantic but also political. Campos has been quick to point out that the International Obesity Task Force that was fundamental to the designation of overweight and obesity cutoff points is funded in part by pharmaceutical companies that sell diet drugs. The hysteria generated around obesity, created in part by the focus on measuring it, he claims, helps to feed both the regulatory passage of and the market for these drugs. For Campos and others, obesity is an acceptable and normal part of human variation that has become improperly pathologized, especially in the twentieth century. The argument goes that weight should be viewed much as height is, and people who are larger than most should no more be expected to change themselves than those who are shorter than most.

One way to view this issue is through the lens of medicalization, the idea that a condition is defined as a disease or requires surveillance but that the definition is more reflective of social context than of biological reality. Culture defines what is normal and hence what is diseased or sick. In other words, "the definition of a specific disease and associated social expectations often depend as much on the society and culture as on the biological characteristics of the disease itself. People labeled as having a particular disease learn 'how' to have it by negotiating with friends and family as well as with people in the treatment system; this process is affected by society's beliefs and expectations for that disease" (Waxler 1998, 147).

In Western societies quite recently, obesity has become highly medicalized, but this is not the case everywhere or historically. In the nineteenth century and earlier, doctors generally felt that carrying an extra 20, 30, 40, or even 50 pounds of weight was healthy, providing vitality and a cushion in the event of severe illness. From the 1870s, a common diagnosis in Western medicine was neurasthenia, or nervous exhaustion, thought to result from mental overwork and indexed by a skinny body with insufficient energy stores. Inactivity and eating were prescribed until the body was larger and thus stronger (Pool 2000, 22).

The recent medicalization of obesity is tightly tied into, rather than distinct from, moral and religious ideas about obesity. Much of the language in the public arena about obesity gives this sense of chaos and crisis. Sobal (1995, 1999) made the point early that concern about the "epidemic" of obesity is a sure sign of its medicalization. The increasing discoveries of a genetic component to obesity (mostly around weight gain) in the last few years will certainly also continue to underwrite its medicalization.

Interestingly, insurance companies, not the medical profession, initiated the medicalization of obesity. In Victorian society, medical notions of weight were related to the need for health and regular appetite rather than to thinness. In the 1920s and 1930s, the medical profession's explanations of obesity tended to favor the "metabolic" causes, such as overweight being a function of glandular or metabolic problems. Actuarial tables, which showed shorter life spans among heavier life-insurance clients, drove a proliferation of obesity-related medical research after the 1930s. The idea of fatness as a widespread and appreciable medical problem appears to particularly emerge after the 1940s, along with the shift from concern from infectious to chronic diseases (lifestyle diseases such as cardiovascular disease, diabetes, and cancer). As Pool points out, the labeling of some overweight cases as "glandular" or "metabolic" and hence beyond the control of the patient, and other cases as the result of the patient's inability to practice self-control, emerged in medicine at that time and persists into the present.

> The endogenous-exogenous distinction provided a useful way of categorizing different types of weight problems, but it also created an artificial dichotomy that shaped thinking about obesity for decades. Now the overweight must be diagnosed as one or the other—responsible or not responsible, shameless or blameless. According to this dichotomy, anyone who is not a victim of a metabolic malfunction must be lazy or gluttonous or both. (Pool 2000, 27)

Global Trends

This notion of obesity as a medicalized condition suggests we might question whether obesity is a disease in its own right, but as we shall see in the next chapter, this model fails to recognize that changes and variation in fat levels have important adaptive, not just medical, implications. Furthermore, this thinking simplifies what is in fact a much more interesting and complicated story about why some people are fat and others are not, playing out at the intersection of the local and the global. It also ignores our short- and long-term

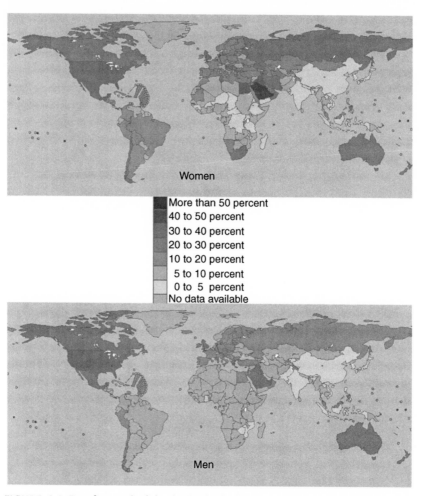

FIGURE 2.3 Prevalence of adult obesity by body mass index (BMI), based on data reported to the World Health Organization at the end of 2009 (WHO 2010).

histories as uniquely cultural beings, which we will explore in more detail in the chapters ahead. However, it does allow us to talk in more informed ways about how obesity risk is distributed globally, because all public health discussions understand the basis for how obesity data are used.

A good starting point for examining how obesity is currently distributed across countries is the World Health Organization's regularly updated database. The current ranking and estimates for all reporting countries are given in appendix A and mapped in figure 2.3. A number of interesting initial observations can be made. One is that, although popular and press discourse sometimes suggests otherwise, Americans are not the most overweight people in the world (although they rank nearer the top than the middle). A list of overweight levels by country that WHO compiled using 2005 data shows that eight of the top ten overweight countries are small nations in the central Pacific. The United States and Kuwait, an oil-rich constitutional monarchy in the Persian Gulf, round out the top ten. Using obesity instead of overweight, the same basic picture emerges: the highest levels of obesity occur in quite different types of places—moderate or poorer but rapidly modernizing Pacific Island nations (Tonga, Samoa, and Nauru), followed closely by the oil-rich Gulf countries of Saudi Arabia and United Arab Emirates, and then by a mix of Western countries led by the United States and the United Kingdom, closely trailed by Mexico, the fattest country in Latin America.

Furthermore, obesity is not confined to any specific countries or regions (or culture groups), and at least some level of obesity is now evident in most countries. Nauru, the United States, and Saudi Arabia have very different cultures, ethnicities, lifestyles, economies, and ecologies. The only thing that links them in any tangible way is a relative absence of people engaged in subsistence agriculture. Compare this scenario to that of countries at the bottom of the lists, such as India and Gambia, where most people still live rurally and off the land. Thus, viewed globally, *where* you live makes a big difference to your chance of being overweight. There is a greater chance of your being overweight if you live in the United States (74 percent) than if you live in Ethiopia (4 percent), where many people are still living rurally and farming, and food shortages are common. Given the diversity of countries in the top third for obesity, though, such singular or simple explanations for why people are becoming fatter globally are insufficient, because countries are so different in terms of biology, history, and economics, as well as culture. In the countries in the middle of the list, in particular, there can be enormous variation in body size, with large sections of the population underweight and large sections overweight, such as in Guatemala, where stunting is widespread (Jehn and Brewis 2009).

Among recent trends in global obesity are these:

- In the developing world, obesity until recently was mainly a condition of educated urban women, but now it is increasingly impacting less-educated women and educated men.
- The only remaining region without noticeable growth in the risk of child obesity in recent years is sub-Saharan Africa.
- Rates of obesity in Latin American, North African, and European transition economies are nearing rates in developed countries.
- Women tend to be more overweight in low- and middle-income countries, while men are more at risk in developed countries.
- Obesity in poorer developing countries and among the very poor in industrialized countries is increasingly associated with reduced height.

- In middle-income countries, rates of obesity are rising fastest among the poor, especially the urban poor.
- While urban dwelling has been associated with greater obesity risk, the gap between rural and urban seems to be shrinking; the rural population is starting to get fatter.
- As middle-income countries rapidly urbanize and industrialize, we are observing more individuals who are underweight or stunted from poor nutrition and more who show signs of overweight and obesity, a particularly troubling trend.
- The obese are getting more obese, especially in industrialized economies; there is now huge growth in the numbers and prevalence of the extremely obese (BMI>40).

Great variation within many countries (including the United States) also makes the national figures a little misleading as a way to understand how risk is distributed. For example, in the United States and increasingly in many other places, minority groups tend to be at greater and increasing risk for obesity. There is also a very complicated relationship between global and local economics and changing average body sizes, which intersects with ethnicity and minority status to create quite a large variation in obesity rates within certain countries (see chapter 4).

Temporal Trends

Regardless of how obesity is distributed within and across countries, risk of obesity has shown a massive increase over the last several decades in almost all parts of the world except sub-Saharan Africa, where obesity rates are steadily increasing despite severe food shortages. This recent and continued upswing in the rates of obesity does not mean that there was no obesity in earlier human history, but rather that until recently the conditions that allowed it to occur were extremely rare. The so-called Venus figurines of prehistoric Europe, dated to more than 20,000 years ago, appear to depict obese female bodies with large, pendulous breasts, thick abdomens, and expansive hips. There is no way to know for sure, but some take the existence of these figures to be clear proof that obesity was a known phenomenon at that time, although it cannot have been common, and it probably occurred only in the most powerful, unusual, or socially fortunate individuals. Written accounts of extremely obese individuals date back to the start of the last millennium in Europe; among the obese were William the Conqueror, Henry VIII, and Louis VI. But until the later part of the twentieth century, obesity was aberrant or highly unusual, and even where it did occur, it was mostly limited to complex societies and to the rich and powerful, who had enough resources at their disposal to eat well all the time.

The spread of obesity globally has happened rapidly and continues apace in most countries. The increases started earlier in the West than elsewhere. The Centers for Disease Control reports some 15 percent of Americans obese in 1980, and more than double that figure by 2006: 33 percent for men and 35 percent for women. In 1990, none of the U.S. states reported obesity rates above 15 percent, whereas by 2007 none except Colorado reported rates under 25 percent. Once considered problems only in higher-income countries, overweight and obesity are now dramatically on the rise in low- and middle-income countries, especially in urban settings.

Currently, the most rapid increases in adult obesity and overweight are occurring in middle-income nations, such as China and India (Monteiro et al. 2004). The quick rise in obesity in middle-income countries reflects the speediness of urbanization, modernization, and entry to global markets. In the poorest nations, such as those in sub-Saharan Africa, where food shortages and undernutrition remain massive problems, obesity is mainly seen in urban and educated women (Martorell et al. 2000). But in China, the effects of rapid income growth mean that overweight risk is growing most rapidly among the less wealthy and less educated sectors (Du et al. 2004). For example, obesity doubled among women and tripled among men from 1989 to 2000 in China (Popkin 2008).

Significant increases in childhood obesity have emerged more recently and are currently growing even faster than those for adults in Western countries. Over the past three decades, childhood obesity in the United States has more than doubled in children ages two to five years, and more than tripled among six- to twelve-year-olds (Institute of Medicine 2005). Some 10 million children over the age of six in the United States are currently estimated to be obese, and the numbers (and proportions) are expected to keep growing.

In the parlance of human biology, a secular trend is a change in average growth patterns that accumulates across generations. After World War II, the major secular trend in many parts of the world was increasing height (as food sources became more abundant and stable). The major secular trend globally now is pronounced weight gain in the absence of increasing height—that is, a trend toward overweight and obesity. The percentage of people in the overweight category has not changed much since 1976 (around one-third of the population), but the percentage of adults classified as obese has increased remarkably (from around 15 to 35 percent of all adults; see table 2.6).

There is some question about whether and if the rapid increase in overweight and obesity, in the United States at least, will continue apace or not. One projection estimates that by the year 2015, 75 percent of adults will be overweight or obese, and 41 percent will be obese (Wang and Beydoun 2007). However, there is also the possibility that the rate of adult obesity in the United States is starting to plateau at around one-third of adults. After twenty-five years

TABLE 2.6

Age-adjusted Percentage of Overweight, Obesity, and Extreme Obesity among U.S. Adults 20 to 74 Years Old, 1971–2006

Weight status	1971–1974	1976–1980	1988–1994	1999–2000	2001–2002	2003–2004	2005–2006
Overweight (BMI 25.0–29.9)	32.3	32.1	32.7	33.6	34.4	33.4	32.2
Obese (BMI ≥ 30.0)	14.5	15.0	23.2	30.9	31.3	32.9	35.1
Extremely obese (BMI ≥ 40.0)	1.3	1.4	3.0	5.0	5.4	5.1	6.2

Source: http://www.cdc.gov/nchs/data/hestat/overweight/overweight_adult.pdf.

of increases, the last few years (2003–2006) have seen some stabilization of the age-adjusted prevalence of adult obesity in the United States at around 34 percent of adults over age twenty, perhaps especially among women, based on one set of national survey data, the National Health and Nutrition Examination Surveys (NHANES). Based on the most recent (2008) NHIS (self-reported) data, the rate of increase has dropped off to almost nothing. The age-adjusted percentage of obese adults in the United States (aged twenty and over) grew from 19.5 percent in 1997 to 25.3 percent in 2005; it was 26.2 percent in 2006, 26.6 percent in 2007, and 26.9 percent in 2008. Nonetheless, it is clear that body sizes will continue to grow in most middle- and low-income countries for some time yet, and the level of childhood obesity will probably continue to rise everywhere, including in the industrialized nations.

3

Obesity and Human Adaptation

An adaptive perspective, which focuses on the process of how human individuals and populations adjust to meet environmental conditions, gives us somewhat different answers than did the preceding chapter to core questions about how much fat is too much. Adaptations are changes by which an organism becomes more suited to its environment; how well an organism is adapted to its environment is referred to as its fitness. An organism's adaptive adjustments can be short or long term, and reversible or not. They range from genetic changes to developmental or technological responses to environmental challenges (Frisancho 1993). This range of adaptive approaches provides several theoretical models that add to our understanding of the social and cultural contexts that embed and shape obesity.

Our species has experienced profound changes during our relatively short evolutionary history, especially with regard to food environments. The diet of our hunting and gathering ancestors over most of the last two or so million years was radically different from the diet of most people now (table 3.1). Until the start of the Neolithic Age some 10,000 years ago when farming lifestyles became prevalent, diets were based on food caught and gathered, such as lean meats, nuts, and fibrous plants. The only readily available drink was water. Since walking was the only way to get around, people likely exercised significantly every day. This "Paleolithic diet" (Eaton and Konner 1985) is arguably the most healthy for our species, since it is the diet our bodies initially evolved to exploit (Cordain et al. 2005; cf. Milton 2002). These foods are barely processed, low in fat (especially saturated fat), high in fiber, and low in sodium; they contain few empty calories. Studies show that modern-day hunter-gatherers are much skinnier and eat much less dietary fat and more fiber than do modern Americans (Eaton and Konner 1985).

TABLE 3.1

**Comparison of Diets of Primates, Contemporary
Hunter-Gatherers, Agriculturalists, and Urban Dwellers**

Wild primate diet[a]	Mainly wild plants of many diverse species with high levels of micronutrients (such as vitamin C); low fat and high fiber intake
Hunter-gatherer diet[b]	Mainly lean hunted meat, supplemented by diverse wild plants
Traditional Polynesian diet	High-quality protein from diverse wild ocean and reef foods (fish and shellfish), starchy carbohydrates from smaller range of domesticated roots and trees, fat mainly from coconut, few wild plants. High fiber, moderate-low fat, nutrient-dense diet.
Modern industrial diet	High level of mass-produced and mass-processed foods high in saturated fat and salt, low in fiber; mostly calorie-dense foods; no wild foods, low levels and diversity of plants, often low in naturally occurring micronutrients (such as iron).

[a] From Milton 2000
[b] From the Ache Indians of Paraguay (Hill et al. 1984)

Seen in this evolutionary context, it is clear that humans essentially put on fat because we are remarkably well evolved to do so. The capacity to store calories as fat conferred an advantage for both survival and reproduction. Fat storage in our species tends to be optimized particularly during pregnancy, childhood, lactation, and illness, when energy demands are highest (Kuzawa 1998; Lieberman 2003). Human reproductive ecologists, who study the human capacity to respond to changing environmental conditions in ways that make biological sense, have shown that extensive exercise and low fat levels on the body can delay or halt ovulation (Ellison 2003). This is the reason many gymnasts fail to ovulate and menstruate at ages that most girls do. Thus, it appears that our reproductive systems have adapted to environmental changes, and these adaptations are mediated by changes in fat stores in interaction with energy expenditure.

The evolved capacity to gain weight when times are good certainly makes adaptive sense for those investing in agriculture, which became a dominant human mode of subsistence 10,000 years ago. Human groups living as subsistent agriculturalists can be particularly prone to seasonal and periodic hunger and to real seasonal variation in energy demands because they often rely on a few key crops. Therefore, weight gain in the food-rich or workload-low times of the year helps to balance out energy demands. For example, for peasant societies, a period of food shortage often comes right before the harvest, and excess calories laid down at other times of the year can compensate during this time. In the rural villages of Gambia, women have significant seasonal swings in weight related to the times when workloads increase dramatically and food availability and quality decline. Gambian women on average oscillate about 5 kilograms (around 10 pounds) in weight, which is about half their total fat stores on average (Prentice and Cole 1994). Some capacity to respond to seasonal cycles in this way is probably fairly normal for our species. Other adaptive strategies observed in subsistence groups in the food-lean seasons, such as reducing workload and other physical activity, may sometimes be invoked rather than using up stored calories (Jenike 1996).

Overall, the regulation of energy stores in humans seems to be both ecologically sensitive and highly efficient. Thus, not surprisingly, when food supplies become constant, it takes little additional caloric input to build large amounts of additional fat on the human body over time. One additional daily Snickers bar, at 273 calories, will add one pound of adipose fat per thirteen days, or nearly thirty pounds in a year (Bray 1987). Over ten years, those Snickers bars would add 300 extra pounds, resulting in morbid obesity.

The spread of obesity in modern environments is thus a product of "stone-agers living in the fast lane" (Eaton, Konner, and Shostak 1988). We are a species designed to live in food environments where sugar is scarce, meat is lean, plants dominate, and the food supply is not always constant and predictable. In contrast, we now live in the midst of cheap, abundant, high-fat, and high-sugar calories. Whereas foods used to require exercise to find or catch, the contemporary diet requires little physical energy expenditure to eat an enormous amount of food. The 10,000 years over which diets have changed dramatically in most parts of the world is insufficient time for major genetic adaptations to our changing food environments. Our biology and our ecology are no longer a good fit.

The Thrifty Genotype

In 1962, James Neel published an extremely influential paper in which he introduced the idea that food shortages during the history of our species led to selection for a more efficient insulin metabolism (Neel 1962). He suggested that this "thrifty gene hypothesis" could explain why diabetes is so common in modern settings, and although Neel's model did not discuss obesity, a number of researchers since have applied his idea to weight gain. In particular, the Neel hypothesis has been applied to understand the very high rates of diabetes and related obesity observed in some Native American and Pacific Island groups in the 1970s through the 1990s.

The basic premise of the thrifty gene argument is that living under hunter-and-gatherer dietary and exercise conditions for millions of years, we evolved a metabolic efficiency that enabled us to survive food shortages but that is not adaptive in our contemporary Western obesogenic environments, where food is always easily accessible. The outcome has been rapid and ubiquitous weight gain in our species (Lieberman 2003). We can thus view morbid obesity and related conditions, such as impaired glucose tolerance and diabetes, as the selective outcomes of an interaction between a thrifty genotype and a comparatively toxic food environment (Wells 2007). One provocative new hypothesis suggests that the metabolic syndrome, which today is associated with obesity and cardiovascular disease, was selected for in our ancestors because it proved a significant advantage for their survival of infectious diseases. The central premise is that fat may have brought about a major improvement in the immune system, thereby protecting overweight individuals in the past from widespread and deadly bacterial infections such as tuberculosis (Roth 2009a). The idea has met with some skepticism from other scientists, who argue that there is no clear evidence that obesity and the metabolic syndrome alter inflammatory responses, and it also does not explain why obesity is increasing so quickly today (Fantuzzi 2009). Roth (2009b) agrees that the evolutionary propositions cannot be properly tested, so the theory cannot be proven.

The thrifty gene model assumes that there must have been some selection for genes that promote weight gain and retention, and that the selection for these genes was probably more forceful in some populations than others. What is known at present about the genetic bases of obesity, and how these genetic variants differ across population groups? A growing body of evidence suggests that there is a genetic susceptibility for obesity and that the heritability of obesity is rather high. For example, one recent study of 5,092 identical and fraternal twins, aged 8 to 11 years, showed that familial association could account for 77 percent of the differences in the children's BMIs and waist circumferences (Wardle et al. 2008). The best evidence for specific genetic variants that can cause obesity are mutations in a single gene (Melanocortin 4-receptor) that is associated with the regulation of feeding behavior. Some 5–10 percent of morbidly obese children have such a genetic variant, which can explain their large-scale weight gain compared to children without the gene variant (Friedman 2003).

The first identified gene variant that codes for relative weight gain in a broad spectrum of the general population was the so-called FTO (fat mass and obesity associated) gene; people with two specific variants of this gene are on average 8.5 pounds heavier, based on a sample of 90,000 people (Loos and Bouchard 2008; Loos et al. 2008). It seems that most of the genes that appear to be related to weight gain are located in the pathways that control appetite, such as control of the brain signals sent by leptin and insulin, which tell us to stop eating. Studies of mice have shown that those without the SH2BI gene are unable to stop eating (Zhiqin et al. 2007).

Does the thrifty gene hypothesis, however, provide convincing evidence for why obesity rates are so much higher in some populations or ethnic groups than others? For example, the thrifty gene concept has been applied to explain why Pacific Islanders, especially Polynesians, have much higher levels of obesity than other groups at the same level of economic development (McGarvey 1994; cf. Allen and Cheer 1996). The hypothesis is that Polynesians may have undergone additional selective events for more efficient metabolism (one that laid down fat more efficiently) during long-distance settlement voyages. Additional fat would have helped them survive cold nights and hunger at sea, and the initial colonization period while waiting for their crops to mature (see, e.g., Houghton 1991; McGarvey 1994). However, this model does not fit well with what we now know about Polynesian navigation and settlement strategies, which probably were sufficiently safe and successful not to constitute a Darwinian event of enough magnitude to select for some survivors in this specific way (Brewis, Irwin, and Allen 1995).

Another case that deserves special attention is the Pima, or Akimel O'odham, Indians of central and southern Arizona. They provide one of the most studied cases of whether the thrifty genotype model helps to explain obesity and diabetes risk. The Pima probably descended from the Hohokam agriculturalists, who fanned out and farmed maize, beans, and squash along the Gila and Salt River drainages, which ran through what is now the Phoenix metropolitan area and surrounding central and southern Arizona. The Pima have for a long time attracted attention because of their very high rates of obesity and associated type 2 diabetes, often described as the highest in the world (Knowler et al. 1990). In the 1960s, the prevalence of type 2 (non–insulin dependent) diabetes was 60 percent among Pima, compared to 6 percent among U.S. whites (Ritenbaugh 1981). The Arizona Pima have thus been the focus of considerable medical effort to find genetic bases for these conditions, with hosts of researchers descending on them over the last few decades.

Mostly, however, these studies have come to naught, with no clear evidence that the Pima are particularly genetically different in ways that would explain their very high rates of diabetes and obesity (Hill 1997; Norman et al. 1998). Many of the Arizona Pima risk factors identified in earlier public health research are those found in other groups—low birth weight, less breastfeeding of infants, relative physical inactivity in both leisure and work time, lower fiber and higher fat diets, and ready access to mechanization and mass-produced food (Dabelea et al. 1999; Kriska et al. 2003; Knowler et al. 1981; Smith et al. 1996). Notably, Pima living a couple of hundred miles south across the Arizona border, in a remote region of the Sierra Madre mountains in Sonora, Mexico, have less than one-fifth the rate of diabetes (6.9 versus 38 percent). Moreover, rates of obesity are one-tenth as common for men and less than one-third as common for women in the Mexican Pima (Shulz et al. 2006).

Anthropologist Carolyn Smith-Morris (2004, 2006) conducted a long-term ethnographic study in the Gila River Pima community, which is home to the majority of the tribe and abuts the Phoenix metropolitan area. She explains how Anglo encroachment of Gila River water and competition with mechanized farming forced a massive change in Pima subsistence patterns around the end of the nineteenth century, with profound, long-term health effects. The move away from farming encouraged sedentism, and the influx of processed food degraded the previously healthy diets. By 1996, some 95 percent of Pima were overweight.

These political economic factors have been amplified in recent years by related cultural and ecological factors. For example, new high-fat dietary items (especially the recently adopted frybread) are important cultural symbols relating to the very notion of "Indianness" and cementing social relations when they are served at gatherings or to guests. In addition, healthy food remains relatively expensive on the reservation, and many Pima are distrustful of medical practitioners. An emphasis is placed on kin networks to maintain health rather than on individual responsibility, and the whole idea of exercise for its own sake is both impractical and culturally foreign (Smith-Morris 2004). The causal bases of high rates of obesity and diabetes among the Pima hence play out in complicated ways across a number of levels beyond the genetic—political, economic, ecological, and cultural. Smith-Morris therefore argues that the only way to create health among the Pima is to focus on comprehensive institutional and social transformation. It is a lesson that likely applies to most other populations as well.

The Pima example illustrates that a newer set of ideas that focus on how fat mechanisms work at the physiological rather than genetic level offer a better way of looking at the biological bases of obesity in relation to differential risks across individuals and populations. The idea of the thrifty genotype—whether selected by disease or by fluctuating food supply—has perhaps had its day and may be best used as a metaphor for framing specific questions about adiposity that can then be tested in the field or lab (McGarvey 1994), rather than as a comprehensive explanation of obesity and diabetes. Newer ideas about how our biology is shaped in the developmental period also move our thinking on this point forward considerably.

The Thrifty Phenotype

Increasingly, human biologists argue that some of the biological variation in our capacity to convert energy to fat (and the related metabolic syndrome) is created by epigenetic effects that occur in utero and in early childhood. Epigenetic effects refer to the interaction of our genotype with environmental factors during development, especially the capacity of a fetus to adjust based on the condition of the mother during pregnancy. Human developmental plasticity tends to deal more quickly, and often better, with rapid environmental changes than does genetic adaptation, in part because the changes can reverse in future generations (Thomas 1998).

The idea of the thrifty phenotype is based on the notion that a pregnant female's body may react to environmental changes in ways that prepare her developing fetus to be better adapted to the world it is entering (Hales and Barker 1992). The mother's nutrition guides this process, a sort of biological "weather forecast" (Bateson et al. 2004) based on maternal condition during pregnancy. Thus babies who are subject to low nutrient supplies in utero tend to develop a lowered metabolic rate, to grow more slowly, and hence to have a smaller body size in adulthood, all of which are good adaptations to living in a world with chronic food shortages (Barker 2001; Bateson and Martin 1999; Gluckman and Hanson 2005). Gluckman and Hanson (2005) call these predictive adaptive responses (PARs). PARs are considered important evolved mechanisms that allow our species to adapt effectively to short-term environmental changes (such as fluctuating food supplies). This model seems to work fairly well explaining generation changes in Pima insulin response (which underlies diabetes), in that birth weights do predict diabetes risk in this group (Lindsay and Bennett 2001).

Although "phenotype" usually refers to the appearance of an organism, such as body size and shape, the term can also refer to the entire physical status of an individual, including function and biochemistry (Gluckman and Hanson 2005). Some aspects of phenotype become fairly canalized or set early in life (such as adult height), but others, such as weight, remain relatively changeable over time. The phenotype in this case refers to a range of developmental plasticities (from very thrifty to much less so) rather than to a dichotomous thrifty versus not thrifty (Wells 2007).

Through most of human history—as hunter-gatherers—there was a good match between what the fetus experienced in utero and the conditions it would experience postnatally. The modal or mean fetal phenotype would have been one programmed in utero to do well under hunter-gatherer conditions, and this would have included depositing fat efficiently when calories were available. However, the thrifty phenotype hypothesis predicts that in developing countries, where fetal growth is more likely than in Western countries to be constrained (by illness or by food shortages), the fetus is much more likely to be at risk for obesity later in life if food becomes readily available, because the fetus is adapted to metabolize calories more effectively.

The thrifty phenotype model also provides a useful and theoretically meaningful way to consider individual differences in our propensity to gain and lose weight as adults, even among people within the same family (Bouchard 2007).

In studies of rats, those that are undernourished in utero are more likely to gain weight on a high-fat diet once born, but also more likely to get fatter on a normal diet (Gluckman and Hanson 2005). It also appears that prenatal environment has the greatest effect on central, abdominal fat, which, as noted, has a high association with chronic disease risk in adulthood.

Thus, the thrifty phenotype hypothesis suggests that people will be more prone to weight gain and retention in adulthood if they were subject to food shortages while they were fetuses and end up living in an environment (like Nauru) where dense calories are always readily available.

Both the genetic and developmental mechanisms for rapid fat accumulation are assumed to have been selected for in the distant human past, when individuals with the capacity to store extra calories efficiently would have been much less vulnerable to environmental food shortages. These selected ecologically responsive developmental mechanisms are thus part of the deeper explanation for the dramatic rise in the rates of the metabolic syndrome and obesity. As Wells (2006, 183) summarizes:

> Early hominid evolution was characterised by adaptation to a more seasonal environment, when selection would have favoured general thriftiness. The evolution of the large expensive brain in the genus *Homo* then favoured increased energy stores in the reproducing female, and in the offspring in early life. More recently, the introduction of agriculture has had three significant effects: exposure to regular famine; adaptation to a variety of local niches favouring population-specific adaptations; and the development of social hierarchies which predispose to differential exposure to environmental pressures. Thus, humans have persistently encountered greater energy stress than that experienced by their closest living relatives during recent evolution. The capacity to accumulate fat has therefore been a major adaptive feature of our species, but is now increasingly maladaptive in the modern environment where fluctuations in energy supply have been minimised, and productivity is dependent on mechanisation rather than physical effort.

The prenatal environment is affected by factors besides maternal food availability. There is accumulating evidence that hormone-mimicking pollutants called obesogens, which are ubiquitous in today's environment, may act on a developing fetus's genes to turn precursor cells into fat cells (Grün and Blumberg 2006, 2009). The result is that an individual's body stores calories as fat rather than burning them, and a fetus programmed to make more fat cells will continue to have these after birth and throughout life. Moreover, the increase in fat cells alters appetite, so the person not only has more fat storage capacity but also gets hungry more often.

Human Biocultural Adaptability

Humans as a species are especially adept at continuously reshaping their adaptive contexts through social and technological innovation and its spread. A useful way to conceptualize this aspect of the adaptive process is via niche construction, the idea that humans seem prone to modify their niche and thereby their adaptive environment, and hence their evolutionary pathways. Humans have massively reconstructed the adaptive contexts in which we now live—through building completely new ecosystems (like cities) that change our capacity to access food and our physical workload, and by developing complex political-economic systems that create, store, and distribute massive amounts of food. Niche construction, because it fundamentally alters the human adaptive environment, can dramatically change human biology and also accelerate natural selection. In this context, obesity represents part of a selection against those poorly adapted to the new, food-rich built environments in which we live. For obesity to be selected against, it would need to be associated with lower reproductive rates or higher risk of death in the reproductive years, which is not instantly evident from the epidemiological studies discussed in the preceding chapter.

The niche construction model suggests that humans may adapt by creating social and ecological solutions to the effects of environmental stressors on human biology. However, social structures can create additional stressors with which we must cope. In this model of adaptation as a process of coping, body size is viewed as a marker for how well individuals or groups of individuals are negotiating their local environments; the patterns of somatic growth thought to be health costly represent the impact of adverse environments on human biology. This model is quite different from one that understands growth outcomes as the result of adaptive tradeoffs. Under the niche construction model, the somatic changes are seen as adaptations, whereas the tradeoffs model considers somatic changes as a potential dysfunction and a reflection of environmental stress and lack of capacity to cope (see Schell and Magnus 2007).

The niche construction model therefore suggests that obesity is an excellent somatic marker of environmental adversity: obese bodies represent the outcome of a process by which individuals and groups "negotiate their environments," not only within the physical environment but also within the webs of social interaction that humans create and in which we are embedded (Crooks, Cliggett, and Cole 2007). The model acknowledges, because people are so diverse, that the "environment" is incredibly complex and the goals of the adaptive process may be contradictory in some cases. This approach allows us to "ask questions about the human organism as a truly bio/social/cultural being" (Crooks, Cliggett, and Cole 2007, 669).

Moffat and Galloway's (2007) study of middle childhood growth in Ontario, Canada, represents a good example of this approach. The authors demonstrate how living in socially disadvantaged neighborhoods creates growth trajectories for children that ultimately put them at much greater risk of obesity than children in environments with better resources and amenities. They compared 266 schoolchildren from three neighborhoods: one very low socioeconomic status (SES) community, one low SES community with higher household incomes and more immigrants, and one high SES community. Using anthropometric measures, the authors show that the low SES children were more than twice as likely to be overweight or obese (34 percent) than the higher SES children (17 percent). They conclude from this study that socially disadvantaged children in low SES neighborhoods are at higher risk of becoming obese or overweight. The high costs of obesity to an individual's health and fertility make it unlikely that what we are observing is an adaptive response; rather it can be seen to represent "local biologies" that reflect the specific adversities with which people are actively coping (Lock and Kaufert 2001).

The ability of some groups or members in a society to exert power over others structures such distributions of risk. Differential distribution of resources accounts for much of the risk, that is, the adverse features of modern environments are not evenly distributed among a society's citizens. However, discrimination itself may also play a direct role (Gravlee 2009; Gravlee, Dressler, and Bernard 2005; Schell 2003).

The niche construction model may also help to explain in part the iterative relationship between poverty and obesity through generations—in other words, the intergenerational effects of the thrifty phenotype. In modern contexts, where large-scale economic and social structures maintain and magnify social inequalities, the constructed niches in which high-status people live are very different from those of low-status individuals. Combining this circumstance and the risks attending the social stigma of obesity (for example, it is harder for the obese to get and keep jobs) explains the action of the intergenerational mechanism beyond genetic or physiological factors. When the effects cycle into the next generation through mechanisms such as low offspring birth weight associated with low maternal status, they can reinforce a "metabolic ghetto, inflicting a deleterious phenotype on the next generation regardless of future environmental conditions" (Wells 2007, 165).

Deborah Crooks's (1998, 2003) research on child growth in rural Kentucky shows how broad political structures (such as school funding decisions) can create these microecologies of risk. Crooks conducted a study in an Appalachian elementary school in the 1990s in a county with high unemployment and underemployment and levels of poverty around 30 percent (double that of the United States as a whole at the time). She found evidence of more variability in growth among girls than among boys, meaning that more girls than boys were at risk of short stature associated with undernutrition (too few calories, too little protein, or both). Boys and girls were both at great risk of being overweight, with 43 percent of boys and 24 percent of girls above the 85th BMI percentile, and 24 percent of boys (but only 8 percent of girls) above the 95th percentile.

Using a combination of ethnographic, anthropometric, and dietary data, Crooks looked at the foods available to children at school, how and why these foods were provided, and the children's overall diets. She found that children were eating snack foods in excess of 750 calories a day, more than a third of the recommended daily intake of calories for them. They ate more than half the snacks at school, and the overweight boys in particular ate more snacks than other children did.

One of the most interesting findings of this study is that administrators at the school understood the nutritional risk of the snacks, but sold the snacks anyway because the sales generated additional money for underfunded school activities such as music, sports, and art. Without the income from snack sales, the children in this lower-resource school district might not have had access to these school activities, and to the administrators "the cost of a less-than-adequate education appears greater than the cost of poor nutritional status" (Crooks 2003, 195).

The model of risk focusing, as explained by University of Albany biocultural anthropologist Lawrence Schell, partly explains how a biological outcome such as obesity might be linked to structural inequities in stratified societies. Risk focusing is the idea that in complex, stratified societies (such as the United States), risk is distributed based on the social, as well as biological, characteristics of individuals (Schell 1997; Schell et al. 2005). A core idea of risk focusing is that negative health outcomes not only result from, but also contribute to, a lack of social or economic advantage (Schell 1992, 1997). Schell's examples focus on lead exposure but might equally apply to obesity. We know that stigma attached to obesity is associated with less job opportunity or less upward mobility, a pattern that would operate in a feedback loop with living in worse neighborhoods with less healthy food environments or fewer exercise amenities. In this model, risk is focused by social and economic forces not only because individuals have several characteristics related to worse outcomes, but also because an interaction between a health outcome (obesity) and risk can be compounded and even accelerated over generations. So, if people who are obese have fewer economic opportunities, and thus are more likely to live in poverty or to be less able to move out from it, and low income also contributes to obesity risk, one could label this loop "transgenerational risk focusing."

In this way, we can start to understand why children of obese parents are more likely to be obese. Not only does risk focusing operate in the children's lives, but also parental obesity contributes to attenuated risk in the next generation, compounding the effect. In other words, for children who are more likely to be overweight because of environmental exposure, weight gain early in life puts them at even greater risk of being obese as adults.

The stress caused by such factors as social exclusion and poverty may also exacerbate these relationships. A growing body of evidence suggests that elevated cortisol, a hormone related to stress and anxiety, can promote the accumulation of fat—especially abdominal fat—as well as underlie greater risk for the metabolic syndrome. The factors that tend to activate the cortisol response in humans include financial hardship, the experience or anticipation of discrimination or prejudice, and depressive and anxiety traits (Björntorp 2001).

One of the useful aspects of risk focusing is that it starts us thinking in bidirectional ways about biology (obesity) and culture relationships; biology not only lies at the substrate of human culture, but also has the capacity to interact with and shape it (Schell 1997). Obesity (a biological phenomenon) might influence culture through its impact on social configuration (for example, by creating a downward movement in social status, either within or across generations), and social configuration may likewise influence obesity. To illustrate, overweight parents have less upward mobility and are potentially stuck in a cycle of poverty to some degree because they are more likely to have and raise overweight children, who in turn have lowered social access to education, employment, and other standard mechanisms for social and economic advancement (Schell 1997). Likewise, adults with low socioeconomic status are at greater risk of obesity, and obesity can then lead to reduced employment opportunities, which in turn leads to lower socioeconomic status. This cycle may pass to the next generation, because overweight adults tend to have overweight children, and early childhood undernutrition and overnutrition are exacerbated by low SES and lead to increased risk of adult obesity.

Thus, risk focusing is a positive feedback cycle: the environmental risks lead to obesity, and obesity leads to increased exposure to the environmental risks that create it (e.g., obesity → lower SES → more likely to live in an obesogenic environment). As Schell (1997, 67) explains:

> Recent studies of biological responses to urban environments and of socioeconomically disadvantaged people indicate that culture allocates risks disproportionately to some individuals and groups within society through its constituent values and related patterns of behavior. Although risk allocation is present in all societies, it is very clear in urban environments within stratified societies where high exposure to harmful materials is many times more likely for some segments of society. In urban environments, culture may be seen as adding stressors to the environment by concentrating naturally occurring materials to levels

that are toxic to humans and through the creation of new toxic materials. In stratified societies the risk of exposure to these new stressors is focused on the socioeconomically disadvantaged. This exposure has consequences that increase the likelihood of more exposure and more socioeconomic disadvantage, thereby increasing social stratification. This suggests that models of biocultural interaction include a feedback relationship in which biological factors influence the sociocultural system in addition to the usual action of the sociocultural system on biological features and responses. This model strongly reinforces the view that stressors can originate from cultural arrangements.

As Crooks, Cliggett, and Cole (2007) have noted in their discussions of undernutrition, these types of biocultural approach raise important questions. How is an obesogenic environment constructed and altered by social actors? What strategies do people develop to deal with those environments? What accounts for the variation in how people engage with and are affected by such environments, and what are the consequences of these different strategies for obesity outcomes? In such biocultural models, culture acts to distribute risk (for example, through differential allocation of resources, including amenities) based on socioeconomic inequalities. Understanding some basics about the social, demographic, and economic patterns of obesity risk in humans can therefore help explain local and global distributions of obesity and suggest potential interventions that could break the feedback loops between socioeconomic factors and obesity.

4

The Distribution of Risk

Until recently, in most parts of the world people lived predominantly on food that they had a hand in growing or collecting, and on foods sourced close to home. The rapid increase in obesity in the United States, other industrialized countries, and increasingly in developing countries during the last three decades is tied to massive and recent changes in our food systems, as well as to a number of highly interconnected factors at the individual, population, and global levels. This macroprocess is often called the "nutrition transition," the term applied to the substantive shifts in diet that have accompanied the global processes of urbanization, modernization, and industrialization. The transition begins when diets rich in whole grains, vegetables, and relatively lean proteins—essentially considered in modern contexts a fundamentally healthy diet—are replaced over time by diets based on more processed foods laden with sugar, saturated fat, and sodium. These dietary changes track associated lifestyle transitions, such as shifts in occupation and leisure-time activities, which tend to promote relative sedentism. Together, these trends explain at a broad level why more people are overweight and obese now than in the past. The rapid pace of these changes indicates that genetic factors are insufficient to explain why so many people are now overweight and obese; social and ecological factors also need attention.

This chapter explores the impact of these macrolevel trends, and also the reasons these massive changes have not affected everyone equally. Many people who live in environments we would classify as obesogenic (ecologies that promote high energy input and low energy output, such as eating big meals, watching a lot of television, and eating food high in fat and sugar) are not overweight. Others who live in food-short environments, such as the shantytowns around large cities in developing countries, are overweight. Recognizing how and why the distribution of risk is so uneven helps explain how and why we need to tackle obesity as a social and political—as much as a health—issue.

48

Given their prominence in the top ten most obese nations, the Pacific Islands make a good starting point to think about the processes that underlie the rapid increase in obesity rates on a global scale. The relatively early rise in obesity in that region compared to other developing countries has brought it scientific attention that generally explains the high level of overweight as the product of modernization over the last several decades. This process includes increasing reliance on imported foods and more sedentary jobs, as these countries have entered the global economy and people have moved away from subsistence farming and fishing to live and work in urban centers (Ulijaszek 2005). (However, bear in mind that not all Pacific nations have extremely high rates of obesity; for example, in highland Papua New Guinea the rates are only around 2 percent.)

Ecological Transformation: The Samoan Case

One of the best-documented cases of the nutrition transition is that among ethnically and genetically similar Samoans living in different areas of the Pacific. Samoan populations have for some time displayed some of the highest levels of adiposity of any human groups (McGarvey 1991). The health impacts of this obesity are reflected in elevated population risks for obesity-related diseases,

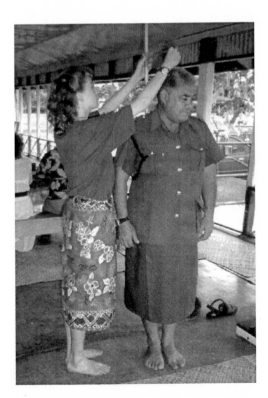

FIGURE 4.1 A student team member measuring the height of the chief of police, Samoa, 1996.

Photo by author.

including cardiovascular disease and type 2 diabetes (Galanis et al. 1995; McGarvey et al. 1993; Zimmet et al. 1981).

Comparing three groups of Samoans helps us understand how the nutrition transition shapes obesity: Samoans in the U.S. territory of American Samoa, those in the nation of Samoa (formerly Western Samoa), and Samoans living in New Zealand. In Samoa and American Samoa, Samoans dominate numerically, socially, and economically. In Auckland, Samoans are a minority immigrant group within a dominant Pakeha (Western) cultural milieu. At the end of World War II, only a couple of thousand Pacific Islanders lived in New Zealand; by 2001 they constituted some 6 percent of the total population.

The Samoans in the three sites vary in diet, occupational and activity patterns, and material item ownership and use (see, e.g., Baker, Hanna, and Baker 1986). In Samoa, far more people produce their own food, far fewer have modern conveniences such as television, and obesity (while not absent) is less common than in the two more urbanized and modernized locations.

For our purposes here, Samoans living in these different settings represent a rough but meaningful gradient of exposure to the influences of modern life (see Baker, Hanna, and Baker 1986), a cross-sectional proxy for a process that has played out over time (see table 4.1). Samoa is classified in this ecological comparison as earlier in the stages of the nutrition transition, New Zealand toward the end, and American Samoa in between—positions that correlate to other factors

TABLE 4.1

Ecological Indicators of Modernization for Samoan Populations, circa 1994

	Samoa	American Samoa	New Zealand Samoans
Samoan % of total population	98	94	5
Women with BMI > 32* (%)	36.3	64.9	55
Women content with body size (%)	45.8	19.3	7.5
Ecological Indicator			
Men in subsistence employment (%)	72	7	0
Households with TV (%)	20	91	97
Mean women's BMI	30.5	35.7	34.1

Sources: Murphy and McGarvey 1994; Brewis and McGarvey 2000.
* Suggested appropriate cutoff for defining Polynesians as obese
(Swinburn et al. 1995)

related to development such as types of occupations, access to cash, and owner-ship of material items. Most parts of the developing world are now well along in the process of the nutrition transition, especially those living in urban areas.

In central Pacific Islands such as Tonga and Samoa, until the 1960s people for the most part ate food they procured or produced themselves, such as coconut, the root crops of taro and sweet potato, breadfruit, yams, bananas, fresh fish, other reef and lagoon foods, chicken, and pork. The traditional diet had few good weaning foods, and most children were fed breast milk well into their toddlerhood. The combination of land and reef resources meant that famine or even food shortages were rare, and—although coconut probably kept their diet higher in fat than is normal for horticulturalists—these islanders gen-erally consumed a fairly healthy combination of high-quality protein and carbo-hydrates (Hanna, Pelletier, and Brown 1986).

In many places around the globe, just as in Samoa, a big part of the nutri-tion transition has been an increasing dependency on imported food and a decrease in high-quality foods such as wild protein, vegetables, and fruits. Over the last century, imports such as flour and white sugar became increasingly noticeable in the Samoan diet, then in many places started to dominate it. Delicacies imported from places like New Zealand and Australia increased, including tinned corned beef, white rice, and turkey tails and mutton flaps (both with 80 percent of calories from fat). All these items have become central to diets in places like the islands of Kiribati and are now highly culturally val-ued. In Kiribati between 1964 and 2001, diets went from an estimated average of 2,159 kcal/day per capita to 2,922 kcal/day, which is in line with dramatic increases in (and growing reliance on) imported foods (Ulijaszek 2005).

In Samoa, as in many other developing countries, urban dwellers are much further along in the nutrition transition than those living rurally, and as a result they are generally more likely to be obese. In cities, people are much more likely to work in the cash economy, have more sedentary jobs, and have greater access to food items (many of which are not particularly healthy). The demands of city life combined with the relative ease of access to prepared, unhealthy foods may make it harder to make time for shopping, preparing, and cooking healthy food at home. These changes are all tied to macrolevel economic trends that trickle down to change the economy in which households make their decisions.

The Dual Burden

The Samoans are different, however, from the many developing countries that entered the nutrition transition with very high rates of undernutrition, often related to periodic famine. In such places, the change to a more Western diet prior to the start of the nutrition transition resulted in an increase in stature, because of the inadequate nutrition of their previous diet. In the Pacific, no such change in stature occurred, which indicates the adequacy of diets pretransition. In many developing countries, especially middle-income nations, it is becoming apparent that the secular trend in weight gain often runs ahead of height increases, and that the causal bases of obesity may be complicated by the simultaneous presence of food shortages and undernutrition. In such countries, more households include both underweight and overweight people (Doak et al. 2005; see also Popkin 1994). A preliminary analysis of survey data for six middle-income nations showed that between 22 and 66 percent of households had both an underweight and an overweight member (Doak et al. 2005).

This happenstance is sometimes referred to as the dual burden of malnutrition, where individuals are simultaneously at risk of obesity and at risk of being stunted or wasted because of lack of food. While this may sound counterintuitive, it makes sense when considered across the life span of an individual. Children who have limited nutrients during their growing years tend to compensate by growing less and end up shorter (an adaptive pattern of growth under adversity referred to in the preceding chapter). If they are later exposed to many nutrient-poor calories (such as when they move to the city or enter the cash economy), they can become obese and are at even greater risk, having less height on which to distribute the new weight (Frisancho 2003; Hoffman et al. 2000). In light of developmental adaptation, permanent changes to metabolism may be associated with undernutrition in early life (such as a preferential metabolic use of carbohydrates rather than fat when energy is required [Frisancho 2003]), which means that excess calories later are more likely to be laid down as fat.

A study that Sarah Lee and I conducted with children living in the shantytowns around Xalapa, Mexico, illustrates this phenomenon (Brewis and Lee 2010; Lee and Brewis 2009). Xalapa lies about five winding hours by bus from Mexico City, up and over the Sierra Madre Oriental Mountains, in a temperate, lush, coffee-growing zone that extends down toward the Gulf of Mexico. As a regional center, Xalapa has attracted campesinos (many unemployed coffee farmers) from the surrounding countryside over the last two decades. In search of new opportunities, these peasant farmers have moved into makeshift towns around the city core. Adults in these communities work in market stalls, factories, and intermittent construction, or in cleaning, seasonal farming, or taxi driving. Household food shortages are common, although families are almost always able to provide at least a basic supply of corn tortillas regardless of circumstances. In poorer homes and lean times, these often have to be made by hand to save money, and there are few luxuries, such as milk or meat, to go with them.

Our project focused on how eight- to twelve-year-old children in these very low income neighborhoods accessed food independently, and how that shaped their nutritional risk. Overweight is rare in this set of children; only 6.3 percent reach the 85th percentile of weight-for-height. Also, unlike the often-overweight upper-middle-class children in the same town I had measured a couple of years earlier, there was no difference in body size between the girls and the boys. More than half the children were stunted (short height-for-age), generally a sign of chronic undernutrition. However, when we look at the diets of these children more closely, we can see how childhood circumstances may set the stage for obesity risk later.

Many of these children were working hard outside the home to earn extra money—running errands, bagging groceries, or helping with construction. In most cases, children got to keep the money they earned, and they used almost all of it to buy extra food—virtually all unhealthy, calorie dense but low in nutrients (for example, chips, sweet drinks, and cookies). In many cases, these items appeared to be replacing lower sugar, lower fat, less-processed foods (mainly tortillas) that they were served at home. Children who did not work for money also often got access to these foods through the common practice of sharing with close friends and younger siblings. Overall, the children who earned money outside the home had worse dietary quality (higher saturated fat, higher empty calories) than those who did not, even when caloric levels were about the same.

The dual burden of malnutrition is not limited to the developing world but occurs, for example, among some very low income populations in North America. Despite the huge increase in obesity, food insufficiency remains an issue in most developed nations, especially those with a large gap between rich and poor. In the United States, for example, in 2007 it was estimated that 36.2

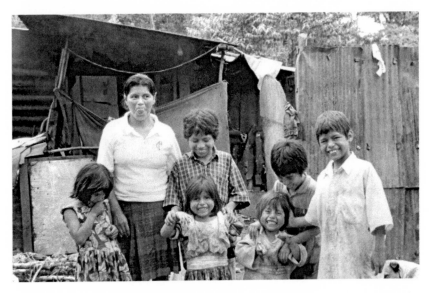

FIGURE 4.2 A dual burden household in Xalapa, Mexico, includes an overweight mother and stunted (short-height-for-age) and underweight (low-weight-for-age) children, 2005.

Photo by Sarah Lee.

million people lived in food-insecure households, lacking regular, predictable food supplies of any quality (Nord, Andrews, and Carlson 2008). One recent study that tracked children in Quebec, Canada, between 1998 and 2002 found higher BMIs in food-insufficient households (those where mothers reported that the children had gone without food or not eaten adequately at least occasionally because food or money had run out), especially among children who had low birth weights (Dubois et al. 2006). Similarly, in a sample of 677 children of seasonal migrant workers from Latin America living in New Jersey, rates of both growth stunting (caused by undernutrition) and overweight well exceeded rates for children in the United States more generally, especially among the boys (Markowitz and Cosminsky 2005).

The co-occurrence of over- and undernutrition is part of the reason that obesity as a biocultural phenomenon can be quite different in developing versus developed countries, as well as between higher and lower socioeconomic status groups within countries. In developing countries and in poor populations, obesity is a condition associated with lower stature (height), while in developed countries and wealthier populations, it is not. As a consequence, many countries that until recently struggled with famine and severe food shortages have quickly segued into dealing with obesity as a major challenge as well. The dual-burden phenomenon complicates nutritional interventions, such as supplemental feeding and education, given that overnutrition and undernutrition traditionally have been treated as distinct problems of nutritional stress with different causative pathways.

Gender and Obesity Risk

Gender is a particularly interesting lens for examining the distribution of obesity risk, because men and women live in the same places globally, including the same homes, but usually have quite different patterns of risk across the board and within any specified population. Men and women have slightly different biologies, but their unique social roles, which are subject to different cultural rules and constraints, better explain the variation in gendered risk. The degree and direction of gender differences to a large extent reflect basic cultural ideas about men's and women's roles, bodies, and behavior, a phenomenon reflected by the variance in gender ratios of overweight and obesity from place to place (see figure 4.3).

Viewed globally, women are more likely to be obese than men, but men are more likely to be overweight than women (Mascie-Taylor and Goto 2007). However, the ratios of male to female risk for both overweight and obesity vary from country to country in interesting ways. For example, let's take the most recent, national-level data for the three countries in which I spend the most time. In the United States, 33 percent of women and 31 percent of men were

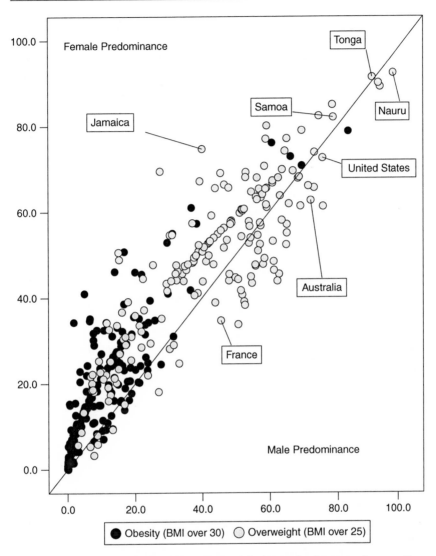

FIGURE 4.3 Ratios of overweight and obese adults by gender for countries reporting data to the World Health Organization prior to 2010. Markers left of the reference line represent countries with a higher incidence of overweight and obese women than of men; right of the line, a higher incidence of overweight and obese men; and on the line, an even gender ratio.

reported to be obese; in Fiji, 24.5 percent of women but only 9.8 percent of men are obese; and in New Zealand, 23 percent of women and 22 percent of men are obese. The highest overweight ratio of men to women occurs in Germany (75.5 percent versus 52.7 percent); in the United States and United Kingdom the ratio is around 70 percent versus 60 percent.

Figure 4.3 presents a plot of the percentage of men and women overweight and obese in all countries where recent data are available through the World Health Organization database. Markers left of the horizontal reference line designate countries where women's weights or BMIs are higher than men's; the further left the marker, the greater the ratio of female obesity/overweight to male. The graph illustrates three interesting points. First, countries vary remarkably in the relative prevalence of overweight and obesity between men and women. Second, in most countries, women are more affected by obesity, and men by overweight, partly a result of men's greater tendency to lay down lean tissue versus adipose tissue when they have excess energy intake. Mostly the scenario is explained by the fact that one cannot be categorized as both overweight and obese, and women overall are heavier. However, in many countries the gender risk is reversed, which is the third interesting point: in some places men are more prone than women to obesity. It is also interesting to consider not only why women are more often overweight and obese (such as the outlier Jamaica), but also under what conditions men might be more at risk in the countries with markers to the right, such as Australia, Germany, and France (the United States and Samoa are both closer to the middle).

Surprisingly little analysis exists from a cultural perspective about how and why women are more at risk for obesity, and why the gender variation shifts as it does from place to place. In epidemiological studies of obesity, most analyses tend to discuss either men or women, not both, or to simply control for gender. In contrast to more explicitly ethnographic studies, there is little focus in the public health literature on the meaning of the variation between the genders in different contexts or the recognition that the variation (because it patterns so differently across populations) must reflect differences in the social construction of gender and gender roles.

I find the idea of developmental niches (sometimes called ecosocial or eco-cultural niches) especially useful for thinking about why men and women who occupy the same households, and presumably have access to the same foods and environmental opportunities for physical activity, can be so differently at risk for obesity. The developmental niche model focuses on how the microinteraction of the psychology of caregivers, customs of child care and rearing, and immediate physical and social settings shape each individual's development. Boys might have very different development environments from girls for cultural reasons, and the physical and social aspects of a niche change with a child's age (Harkness and Super 1994; Super and Harkness 1982). This model is especially useful for thinking about how culturally situated parental child-feeding practices might shape child eating, and also for thinking about how individual-level characteristics (such as age, household composition, or food availability) might be built into our models. Our work in middle-class Mexico, discussed in the preface, that showed male school-children were at much greater risk of obesity compared to their girl peers rested heavily on this idea (Brewis 2008). Gender, as noted, is variably associated with changing obesity risk across populations. In many cultural settings, parents may feed boys and girls differently, mainly because of the value placed on each gender, and also gender-specific ideas about what feeding is appropriate. For example, parents might differently restrict calories for girls and boys if they perceive greater social costs to girls being overweight than to boys. Alternatively, they may feed sons more at the expense of daughters if the growth and survival of boys is more important to the family. Birth order or family configuration also makes a difference in some settings; for example, single children can live in quite different microecologies than those with a number of siblings.

The developmental niche is an example of a model that allows consideration of immediate and proximate culture-individual interactions, as well as of the ecological reactivity of culture (e.g., Harkness and Super 1994; Worthman 1994). In this case, "culture" is often identified mainly as ethnotheories, meaning culture-specific ideas about how the world works; examples include ideas about the right way for a child to be fed and to eat, and about appropriate types of exercise or body shape for women and men. But culture could equally include culture-specific ideas about bodies, such as ideas about what size one should want to be and about what sizes are acceptable. These ideas often differ for girls versus boys or women versus men, given the different social roles each is expected to (or has the opportunity to) occupy. It is also notable that a large body of psychology research has considered the role of children's temperament in shaping these developmental niches, which may have implications for shaping obesity risk. For example, babies with fussier temperaments are more likely to be bottle-fed or breast-fed for a shorter duration, which is a predictor of obesity (see, e.g., VanDiver 1997; also see Wachs 2008).

As noted, our work in an upper-middle-class Mexican school during a study in Xalapa in 2001 used the niche concept to illustrate how gender-specific ethnotheories about appropriate child eating, nutrition, and activity may promote or reinforce gender differentiation in microniches and thereby influence boys' versus girls' likelihood of being obese (Brewis 2003). For the study, we took anthropometric measures (skin folds and BMI) for 110 girls and 109 boys, ages six to twelve years—about half the students in a single school (the number whose parents consented to their participation). We found that more than a quarter of the children were obese (using the 95th percentile as the cut point). The rates were markedly higher among boys (30 percent) than girls (20 percent), and highest among boys who were the only child in their family (over 60 percent).

I was particularly interested in how individual socioecological variation (such as differences in exercise, diet, family, household, parental, and demographic factors) could explain the high rates of overweight in this school, and of boys in particular. Although a number of other studies have since documented rising childhood obesity rates in Mexico, reports of that sort were uncommon at the time. It was difficult to tell if we were detecting the edge of a coming trend (we were, as it turned out) or a discrete ecological phenomenon. I found the idea of developmental niches a helpful way to think through and test hypotheses, because gender could be incorporated as a potentially critical component of each child's developmental niche, for example, how parents treat girls versus boys (Lancaster 1994; Worthman 1996, Worthman et al. 1993), and thereby shape different, gendered bodies.

As we have described elsewhere (Brewis and Schmidt 2003), the parents of these children had a characteristically permissive and responsive parenting style compared to the more authoritarian approaches that have been described as typical of Mexicans (Frias-Armenta and McCloskey 1998). Interestingly, we also found that the risk of obesity was highest among children who had the most permissive parents. Furthermore, the very high emotional value placed on children, especially sons, in smaller, middle-class families could result in indulgent feeding because food treats are a cultural index of parental caring.

This relationship between permissive parenting and overnutrition is not necessarily a generalizable finding (for example, Danish parents' restrictiveness is associated with increased obesity in their children [Lissau and Sorensen 1994]). However, ethnographically and contextually, it is easy to describe how this might happen in middle-class Mexican families. One way these parents indulge their children is with a fairly constant flow of sweet treats and high-fat snacks. Based on informal ethnographic observation, this is most pronounced among working mothers, who showed up at school offering lots of cuddles and candy to their children. The smaller the family, the more attention each child receives, especially because in Mexico food is an index of caring attention.

Furthermore, while these Mexican parents treasure daughters and sons, they award special primacy to male children, especially the firstborn. Olvera-Ezzell, Power, and Cousins (1990) found that Mexican American mothers of boys encouraged their sons to eat more than did mothers of girls. Such a simple cultural mechanism, especially if it was heightened in firstborn or only sons, would be sufficient to explain the gender variation we observed. Notably, parents, even those with technically obese children, did not generally identify their children as having a weight problem. With the number of undernourished children living in Xalapa, such as those in the shantytowns discussed earlier, it is not surprising that parents valued a little chubbiness in their children as a sign of health.

Residence Location and Obesity

Rates of obesity vary markedly from country to country and also across regions, as discussed earlier. Currently, the lowest rates of obesity are in sub-Saharan Africa, where food shortages and famine are still common and economic

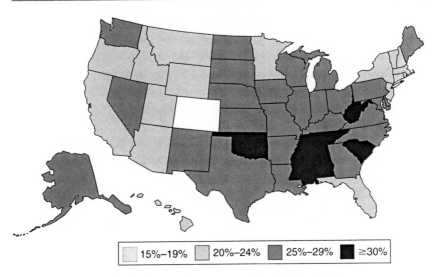

FIGURE 4.4 U.S. adult obesity rates by state, 2008 (see CDC 2008b).

development has been slowest. Within regions, and even within localized areas, location also seems to have profound influence on body size and risk of obesity. In the United States, for example, a significantly higher level of adult obesity occurs in the South and Midwest than in other regions (see figure 4.4). In 2008, thirty-two states had a prevalence of obesity equal to or greater than 25 percent; in six states—mainly in the South (Alabama, Mississippi, Oklahoma, South Carolina, Tennessee, and West Virginia)—around a third of people were obese. Colorado is the only state that had less than 20 percent obesity in 2008. The higher obesity rates in the South are generally explained by cultural values that favor sweet, high-fat foods, and by lower levels of income and education.

With regard to country, place of birth and duration of residence is also important, and is taken to support the environmental hypothesis of obesity. In the United States, members of immigrant groups increase in size and obesity prevalence with time and across generations, meaning the longer they live in the United States, the greater their relative weight gain (see, e.g., Goel et al. 2004; Popkin and Udry 1998). A large study of U.S. adolescents showed, for example, that Hispanics and Asian Americans born in the United States are twice as likely to be obese as individuals in the same ethnic groups who were born elsewhere and immigrated to the United States (Popkin and Udry 1998). This pattern appears in a wide range of studies: even though BMI differs significantly based on country of origin, BMI in the second and third generations substantively increases to match or even exceed the rate of nonimmigrants (e.g., Bates et al. 2008; Himmelgreen et al. 2004; Sanchez-Vaznaugh et al. 2008; Sundquist and Winkleby 2000).

Historically, U.S. rural populations have tended to have much lower rates of obesity overall than their urban counterparts. The initial rapid rise of obesity in urbanizing areas in most parts of the world has been viewed mainly, for people who move to cities, as a function of the dietary changes that result from the relative abundance, cheapness, and processed nature of food available; the move away from rural subsistent and traditional diets; and the adoption of more sedentary lifestyles. However, more recent observations suggest that rates of obesity are also rising rapidly in many rural areas, and the gap between urban and rural is closing.

The relationship between obesity risk and urban versus rural residence is an important one, if only because the majority of humans now live in cities. However, cities are complex places, and lifestyles can vary markedly among their residents, depending on social, economic, and spatial factors. A number of recent studies have attempted to look at more fine-grained patterns of obesity risk in cities, especially differences between neighborhoods. Many of these studies take an environmental approach, relating local risk of obesity to variations in the built environments of various cities and parts of cities (Hill et al. 2003; Poston and Foreyt 1999). For example, local environments such as neighborhoods can be considered obesogenic when they do not provide a structure amenable to or encouraging of physical activity, and as leptogenic (Egger and Swinburn 1997), or causing a reduction in weight, when they are structured in ways that strongly encourage or even demand physical activity.

This distinction is particularly pertinent in suburban and inner-city areas, where different built-environment configurations can have dramatic effects on how residents exercise in their day-to-day lives. For example, parts of Manhattan encourage walking: it is easier to get around on foot than by car, and many people forgo owning a car because of features of the built environment, such as easy access to public transport, lack of parking, and easy foot or bicycle access to places they want to go. In contrast, in many U.S. cities such as Los Angeles and Phoenix, it is difficult to get anywhere without a car, because of the large distances between destinations and the relative paucity of good public transportation.

These differences in the built environment are important because, although results differ by age group, the general consensus is that childhood obesity risk declines with access to local opportunities for physical activity (Sallis and Glanz 2006). There is also evidence from the built-environment studies that conventional suburban neighborhoods, with low-density housing, cul-de-sacs, and heavy reliance on cars, tend to be associated with higher BMIs than are more traditional urban and suburban neighborhoods, with their higher housing densities, greater number of connected sidewalks and streets, and less car-friendly nature, which encourages people to walk or bike to do errands (Smith et al. 2008; Saelens et al. 2003).

In our research in Phoenix, we have been focusing on two specific aspects of the built environment: local walkability and park access (Cutts et al. 2009). We think these factors influence how obesity risk is constructed within neighborhoods by differentially influencing leisure-time exercise. In the United States, some 84 percent of the population walks for recreation, making it the most likely and easiest form of leisure-time exercise (USDA Forest Service 2006), and neighborhood streets are the physical spaces in which people most frequently walk (Giles-Corti and Donovan 2002). More walkable neighborhood streets correlate with both higher levels of physical activity and lower BMI (Saelens et al. 2003). A neighborhood with very low walkability is one with unsafe or absent sidewalks (with broken portions, poor lighting, fast traffic, or high crime); is unpleasant to walk in (for example, because of trash or aggressive dogs); or has no desirable destinations for people to walk to (Booth, Pinkston, and Poston 2005; Doyle, Kelly-Schwartz, and Schlossberg 2006; Ewing et al. 2003; Roemmich et al. 2006). In Phoenix, the role of shade is a consideration in the summer, when temperatures can make being outdoors unpleasant and even dangerous. Phoenix neighborhoods with lots of shade from large leafy trees are much cooler than those without shade and those that suffer from a localized heat-island effect because of differences in factors such as vegetation, paved surfaces, and pollution levels.

In considering park access, a particular concern is distance of residences from parks, a major predictor of park use (Boone 2008) along with park facilities (Kaczynski, Potwarka, and Saelens 2008). People who have easy access to urban parks are nearly three times more likely to get the recommended amount of daily physical activity (Giles-Corti et al. 2005), and while the science is a little vague, it is agreed that childhood obesity risk generally declines with better access to local opportunities for physical activity, including green spaces (Sallis and Glanz 2006).

While the physical environment itself is important in shaping risk, people's perceptions of that environment are also critical; if people think that a neighborhood is unsafe or that there is nowhere of value to walk to, they will be less likely to walk (Giles-Corti et al. 2003; Humpel, Owen, and Leslie 2002; Timperio et al. 2005). Similarly, people's perceptions of the quality of parks or other green spaces can sometimes better predict the likelihood they will use them for exercise than can objective park attributes.

Also likely contributing to the creation of obesogenic neighborhoods are food deserts, areas where it is difficult to access fresh, healthy food at a reasonable price. Some rural areas are food deserts, in that one may have to travel some distance to access reasonably priced, healthy food. For example, in Washington-Wilkes County, Georgia, where we did research on child feeding and nutrition, the closest large supermarket was more than twenty miles away. People had to have their own reliable transport to get there, and the opening of this supermarket had forced the closing of a smaller one in the center of town.

Where food deserts have been most often identified, however, is in older, inner-city areas in the United States, Canada, the United Kingdom, Scotland,

and Australia (Whitacre, Tsai, and Mulligan 2009). In many inner cities, especially in areas with lower-income residents, one may find few or widely spaced full-service supermarkets. Residents without means of transport or extra time to shop farther away (as is often the case for the poorest) are more likely to have to shop at convenience or corner stores. These stores typically have less fresh produce, poorer quality produce, and higher prices. They also tend to stock food with long shelf lives, like cookies, chips, and soft drinks, that tend to be highly processed and mass produced, high in corn syrup and sugar, and laden with cheap oil—types of food high in calories and low in nutrients by both weight and price. Such foods are also are more likely to be converted into fat by the body because they metabolize differently from foods such as fruits, vegetables, and wild or free-range meat. Contributing further to the obesogenicity of inner-city environments are the often higher densities of fast-food restaurants, putting unhealthy but very cheap meal choices within a short walking distance.

These environmental factors not only lead to more fast-food consumption but also degrade diets at home, promoting the risk of nutritional morbidities such as obesity and diabetes at the neighborhood level (Gallagher 2006; Horowitz et al. 2004; Morland, Diez Roux, and Wing 2002; Powell, Auld, et al. 2007; Sharkey and Horel 2008; Sloane et al. 2003). For example, a study of 10,000 residents of Maryland, North Carolina, Mississippi, and Minnesota found that residence location had a significant effect on the amount of fruits and vegetables consumed (Morland, Diez Roux, and Wing 2002). Poor food environments include a visual factor, such as bombardment via billboards and other forms of advertising of food images designed to promote consumption.

The idea of food deserts as a structural contributor to obesity is catching on among those interested in obesity prevention. In a number of places, community groups and government agencies have been working to attract new supermarket development, restock existing supermarkets, transport shoppers, and support street vendors, farmers' markets, urban gardens, and food cooperatives in order to create "food oases" that will improve the overall health and well-being of communities (DeMattia and Denney 2008; Mikkelsen and Chemini 2007).

Several scholars have raised reasonable concerns that this intervention and prevention is occurring without a sufficient scientific basis for the assumption that better household access to grocery stores (or other affordable healthy food sources) translates into healthier eating (Baker et al. 2006; Cummins et al. 2005; Cummins and Macintyre 2002, 2006; White 2007). The few studies that have directly tested the relationship between food environments and what people eat report mostly contradictory or modest results (Morland, Diez Roux, and Wing 2006; Powell, Auld, et al. 2007; Powell, Slater, et al. 2007; Rose and Richards 2004; Smoyer-Tomic et al. 2008; White 2007; Wrigley, Warm, and Whelan 2002). Needed at this juncture is clarification of whether food access independently predicts dietary intake (White 2007) in a way that ties individuals and their households to neighborhood-level effects (Ford and Dzewaltowski 2008). Social processes, such as people finding socially based solutions (food sharing or car pooling) to the challenges of adverse food environments, may help to explain the ambiguous findings to date.

The upshot of all this is that our risk of obesity is probably influenced in myriad structural ways by neighborhood food and exercise environments. If you live in a safe, dense neighborhood with easy access to wonderful parks, fresh healthy food sources, minimal junk food, and desirable places to walk to, you are less likely to be overweight because the environment in which you live encourages you to make healthier choices on a day-to-day basis. Current research supports this connection, although it is mainly based on cruder, population-level associations between built-environment characteristics and BMI levels or obesity rates. Better longitudinal studies that link environmental changes (such as the entry of new supermarkets) to change at the household and neighborhood levels are needed to confirm the science (Cummins and Macintyre 2006). Also, notably, these food desert studies have to date largely been conducted in cities in the United States, England, Scotland, Australia, and New Zealand. We do not know whether the situation is similar in the urban areas of developing countries. However, we might expect that as cities in developing countries move through the nutrition transition, some of the same patterns might occur, in that worse food and exercise environments will tend to be found in areas where the poor or minorities are located.

Socioeconomics and Obesity

The complicated but fundamental relationship between income, economic and social standing, poverty, and obesity deserves careful attention. It also helps us in part unpack the relationship between deprivation, obesity, and ethnicity, important for understanding how culture and obesity are linked.

In 1989, Sobal and Stunkard published an influential review that summarized the findings of 144 studies spanning the 1960s to 1980s from a wide range of countries that examined the relationship between obesity and socioeconomic status (SES). They found that developing-country women, men, and children of higher SES were more likely to be overweight than those of lower SES. In developed countries, they found either the reverse or equivocal results for women. For men, about half the studies found a positive relationship between SES and obesity, and about half an inverse relationship. The results for children were also not consistent.

The basic patterns suggested by the 1989 review have been reinforced by studies since. In low-income countries, the higher the SES, the larger the person. In high-income countries, the higher the SES, the smaller the person. And in countries making the transition between low and middle income, where income gaps are growing and populations are rapidly urbanizing, the risk of obesity is shifting down the SES ladder, toward the urban poor in particular.

Monteiro and colleagues (2004) documented the spread of obesity to lower SES groups in developing countries between 1989 and 2003. In particular, there was a shift toward increasing risk in low SES groups that took place sooner and to a greater extent for women than men, with the tipping point a GNP of around $25,000 per capita.

McLaren in 2007 classified individual countries into three categories based on their UN-assigned Human Development Index (HDI), which ranks countries based on factors such as life expectancy, standard of living, and gross domestic product. Germany, New Zealand, and the United States are high-HDI countries; of the middle-HDI nations, Brazil and Saudi Arabia are at the high end, Nauru is in the middle, and Kiribati is at the bottom; Burkina Faso and Haiti are low HDI. McClaren found that for women in high-HDI countries, obesity was associated with lower SES. In low-HDI countries, the relationship between obesity and higher SES in women remained. Middle-HDI countries presented mixed findings. (Mostly, these studies used education as a proxy measure of SES.) For men in high-HDI countries, there was either no perceptible relationship between SES and obesity, or the risks were highest in high-, low-, or middle-SES men. For medium-HDI countries, the results were similar, but the second-most-common pattern was a positive rather than a negative association. The three studies in low-HDI countries all showed higher SES associated with greater prevalence of obesity in men.

Overall, a comparison of Sobal and Stunkard's and McLaren's analyses suggests a closing of the SES gap. In particular, high-income women in high-income countries do not have the propensity to relative thinness observed in the past. McLaren concludes that although high-SES women in high-income countries may still value and pursue thinness, the "widespread and relatively non-discerning nature of the current obesity epidemic" (McLaren 2007, 33) shows that social groups are no longer immune to the pervasive nature of obesogenic environments. However, she notes that the inverse relationship between SES and obesity is still evident, at least among women in high-HDI countries.

Baseline obesity levels have risen within countries almost across the board as per capita gross domestic products (GDPs) have risen. However, there is no simple relationship between a country's per capita GDP and obesity rate. There are also plenty of outliers—high-GDP Japan has low obesity rates. (Japanese diets are much healthier than those in other industrialized nations, and the high cost of automobiles contributes to more walking in daily life.) It has for some time been recognized that complicated relationships exist between the social and economic standing of societies, individuals within those societies, and level of obesity.

Further, socioeconomic status is a complicated concept that attempts to encapsulate complex information about a person's life relative to that of others (Blane 1995). SES is widely invoked not only in obesity research but also in health research more generally, because it tends to highly predict a lot of health outcomes. However, no generally accepted definition or standard exists for its measurement (Oakes and Rossi 2003); usually, the measurement of SES uses some combination of individual or household income, education, and occupation to estimate relative economic and social position.

There have been efforts to figure out which aspects of SES might best predict obesity risk, which for one thing would help shape better interventions. Level of education is a regularly cited determinant of obesity risk, although it is often used as a proxy for or considered highly associated with socioeconomic status. In developed countries, it is accepted that the incidence of overweight is greatest among disadvantaged groups, which also seems to be the case in middle-income countries. Similarly, Mendez and Popkin (2004) present evidence that in urban areas of highly urbanized countries, women of low SES (as measured by education) are more likely to be overweight than those of high SES, whereas the reverse is true in countries with low urbanization. It seems probable that urbanization in this context is really a proxy for income and socioeconomic status (all correlate highly).

At the most basic level, over time we might expect the relationship between rising income and obesity to begin as a positive one, then reverse at some economic tipping point when cheap, easy access to food is guaranteed but the social costs of excess weight become intolerable. The empirical evidence supports this scenario fairly well. For example, a recent analysis comparing a range of countries found that BMI in women peaks at about US$12,500 purchasing power parity (PPP) and in males at US$17,000 PPP (Ezzati et al. 2005). Trail (2006) explains the cognitive tradeoff in economic terms:

Assuming that everyone has an "ideal" body weight—a weight that they would like to be for reasons of health and/or appearance, and that they would aspire to if it did not cost them anything to achieve in terms of money, effort or foregone pleasure from eating and drinking less than they would like—people whose weight is below their ideal would use some or all of any increase in income to eat more; for such people, weight increases with income and they derive extra utility both from eating and from being closer to their ideal weight. Weight will also be positively related to income for people who are heavier than their ideal weight, as long as the additional pleasure derived from being able to consume more food (and drink) exceeds the loss in utility from any extra weight they would gain. However, beyond some point, the losses in utility from gaining weight exceed the increases in utility from eating more, and the people affected are no longer prepared to spend more of their incomes on a greater quantity of food. In fact, there are good reasons to expect that as such people's incomes continue to increase they will spend money to be less overweight if they can, by buying more expensive healthy foods, joining gyms, paying for membership of weight-loss groups, etc. The relationship between income and weight is therefore predicted theoretically to be positive at first, then negative—although most people choose to be somewhat overweight.

A number of studies conducted in the United States have shown how complicated the associations between income or SES and obesity can be. Overall, lower SES is associated with higher weights by height and increased risk for obesity within the major ethnic groups in the United States (e.g., Scharoun-Lee et al. 2009). The relationship between obesity and SES is apparent among adolescents who identify themselves as white but not, however, among those who identify as African American or Mexican American (Gordon-Larsen et al. 2003). And it appears that obesity is growing particularly fast in the United States in higher income brackets, while National Health and Nutrition Examination Survey (NHANES) data show declining disparities in obesity risk as it relates to wealth during the last two decades (Wang and Beydoun 2007). Moreover, the strong relationship between SES and obesity once thought to exist in the United States may be weakening (Wang and Zhang 2006). Basically, the disparity is declining because more people are growing fatter across the board, not because the situation is improving.

A range of studies from middle- and high-income countries, including the United States, England, Brazil, and Japan, have clearly shown an inverse relationship between education level/socioeconomic status and obesity rates. That is, higher obesity is observed in the lowest-income sectors of societies.

The Dual Burden and Other Complications

The relationship between poverty and obesity is further complicated by the dual burden of malnutrition discussed earlier. Anyone who has spent time with poorer urban families in the developing world is likely to have seen cases of this convergence of overweight with underweight all around them. For example, in the Mexican urban shantytowns where we recently completed a study of children whose families had migrated from the countryside, it was not uncommon to find a family with a mother who was stunted, anemic, and overweight, a husband who had a normal weight but high blood pressure, and a child who was undernourished.

Particularly for the poor, and most especially in the middle-income countries, we see the dual-burden phenomenon exploding. That is, poverty is creating pathways to both undernutrition and overnutrition that attenuate the negative effects of both. The spread of the dual burden seems tightly tied to economic changes both at the national and household level. Data from China, Brazil, Indonesia, Kyrgyz Republic, Russia, Vietnam, and the United States show that the prevalence of the dual-burden household (one with both underweight and overweight members) tends to increase with economic development in the poorer and middle-income countries (although sometimes it is associated with wealthier sectors of low-income areas) and is more common in urban settings (Doak, Adair, Bentley, Zhai and Popkin 2002; Doak, Adair, Bentley, et al. 2002; see also Kapoor and Anand 2002). Garrett and Ruel's (2005) standard regression analysis indicates, however, that urban residence outside the Americas is not necessarily predictive of the risk of a stunted child having an overweight mother, although economic development (defined as per capita GNP) is predictive in this way. Thus, at present the dual-burden household is proposed as a corollary of relative economic development and more generally of the nutrition transition, whereby as national income rises in the poorer nations, changes in diet and activity patterns increase the risk of overweight and obesity, while many of the risk factors for undernutrition remain.

However, the economic contexts that explain the emergence of dual forms of malnutrition at the more local (individual, household) level and how this proximate risk articulates with broader shifts in national and regional wealth are poorly understood. Studies examining local-level data are limited in geographic scale, and many highly correlated variables (such as urban residence, employment type, education, and household wealth) are not disentangled (Angeles-Agdeppa, Lana, and Barba 2003; Florencio et al. 2001; Khor and Sharif 2003; Raphael, Delisle, and Vilgrain 2005). Collectively, these studies suggest that urban residence, maternal education, and maternal occupational standing are proximately important in explaining the collision of risk for under- and overnutrition. In a summary overview, Caballero (2005) posits that urban marginal poverty might provide a particular locus for coexisting paradoxical forms of malnutrition because migrating families lose the ability to grow their own food, and mothers increasingly working to support the family are doubly dependent on cheap, commercially prepared food. He also identifies access to television, particularly where it is not balanced with better nutritional education, as another risk factor.

Epidemiologist Megan Jehn and I recently used demographic data collected by the USAID to better evaluate the influence of various aspects of social and economic standing within and across studies to determine how this risk becomes manifest (Jehn and Brewis 2009). We were concerned with better understanding which proximate economic and socioecological conditions are the causal pathways to undernutrition and overnutrition, how they are most likely to converge, and how these relate to household poverty in countries with different levels of economic development. To do this, we combined very large samples with a model that allows for a range of covariates, so that we could identify with greater precision how variation in ecological and economic circumstances might be merging risks for underweight and overweight within households.

Our analysis focused on identifying overweight mothers with underweight children as our marker for paradoxical (dual-burden) households. We used data from households in low- and lower-middle-income countries in four world regions (northern Africa, sub-Saharan Africa, South Asia, and the Americas). We looked at how factors such as relative country wealth, relative household wealth, urban residence, and employment might independently, and in interaction with each other, lead to paradoxical obesity. We used a variety of measures to assess SES, which in this case was really a measure of relative wealth but particularly focused on household material assets.

As have other studies, we found that living in urban areas was associated with paradoxical households (Doak et al. 2000) and with the highest prevalence of both maternal and child overweight, which is consistent with the hypothesis of rapid adverse changes in dietary composition in these areas. In line with existing studies for developing countries, overweight mother/normal weight children pairs were more likely to occur in wealthier households. Our finding that overweight mother/underweight children pairs were less prevalent in less wealthy households is somewhat inconsistent with previous large international studies, especially Doak et al. 2000.

Overall, our results suggest that while the dual burden is observable in many early- and mid-transition developing countries, it might better be understood and addressed in many cases as a byproduct of rapid increases in maternal overweight occurring sooner than, or without changes in the risk of, child undernutrition, rather than as a discrete nutritional condition. That is, the dual burden is a side effect of the rapid transition to overweight occurring in many households as they confront the diet and exercise changes associated with urbanization and globalization.

In summary, the overall process appears to be this: as countries begin and then accelerate economic development, BMI starts to climb. This rise is associated with increasing urban migration, a shift from traditional occupations, increased technology in the workplace and home, and increased articulation with and dependence on the cash economy and global food systems. In the early stages of the transition, BMI increases occur mainly in the wealthier sections of society and undernourishment remains common in other sectors. As the transition proceeds, more people are affected, the proportion of undernourished diminishes, and overall BMI goes up. In the middle of the transition, especially if it is occurring quickly, overweight and underweight tend to converge. By the end of the transition, all sections of society show high risks of obesity, with the greatest risk in the poorest groups. Whereas obesity was once the preserve of the rich, it is now the preserve of the poor—although unless patterns change, it is increasingly becoming an equal opportunity condition.

People can be time poor, as well as money poor; awareness of this phenomenon is important in thinking about associations between income, poverty, and obesity risk. Low- and middle-income households in the industrialized West, and increasingly urban families in developing economies, have to make complicated tradeoffs between how they use their money and their time. Where people have sedentary or fixed-location jobs with long, inflexible hours, time poverty can be a real problem for both eating and exercising. Families in poverty tend to face the most difficult tradeoffs, because their choices are often so comparatively limited. For example, when both parents are working and money is still short, there is less time in the house for sourcing and preparing healthy meals that may require greater shopping effort and preparation time. Shopping for and preparing food from scratch takes effort, and fast food or pre-prepared foods, often high in fat and low in nutritional value, are increasingly the most time thrifty and often the cheapest available calories.

In the United States, the USDA's Thrifty Food Plan, used to determine maximum Food Stamp allotments, suggests the types of foods that people could purchase and prepare on a low budget to provide a nutritious diet. However, these low-cost plans require about sixteen hours per week of food preparation time, well above the national average of six hours per week working women typically spend preparing food (Rose 2007). Families who eat together tend to eat fewer fatty foods and more fruits and vegetables, but the growing norm in working families is to spend less at the grocery store and more at fast-food restaurants and on easy, pre-prepared foods. Technological changes have made a huge supply of affordable, pre-prepared foods available to households, and it appears that in many ways this availability has increased consumption, especially of snack foods (Cutler, Glaeser, and Shapiro 2003). Clearly, exercise also requires a time investment for people with sedentary jobs, if they are to meet the basic health recommendation of thirty minutes of vigorous exercise most days.

Ethnicity, Obesity, and Culture

Although we can (and soon will) critique the idea that ethnicity matters in explaining obesity, it is important for a number of reasons to understand how obesity rates vary by ethnicity. First, ethnicity rates are among the most often reported figures about obesity in the media and in scientific literature. Second, the public and community health and intervention literature increasingly recognizes that the bases of obesity risk might operate differently across ethnic groups.

How much of the correlation between obesity risk and ethnicity is cultural, and how much is due to other factors that covary with race/ethnicity, such as income? For example, statistical analysis of U.S. national-level data shows that obesity risk among Hispanic/Latino individuals increases with both time and number of generations in the United States, and that U.S.-born children of immigrant parents appear the most at risk. This risk is most often explained as a product of greater exposure to the American environment, which creates less healthy dietary and exercise behaviors. However, Latino/Hispanic risk in the United States remains higher than that of other groups even controlling for diet. Thus, recent hypotheses for the elevated risk of Mexican Americans include lower physical activity levels (Crespo et al. 2001), decreased metabolic utilization of fat relative to undernutrition prior to migrating (Frisancho 2003), increased reliance on low-cost, high-calorie food, and elevated caloric intake via sweet drinks (Giammattei et al. 2003).

These findings raise the question of whether Latinos in the United States are more at risk of obesity because of some inherent cultural factor related to being Latino, because Latinos are more likely to be lower income or live in built environments that create risk, or both? The complex issue of the apparent link between obesity and ethnicity concerns culture, but perhaps not in the most obvious senses. The two things we do know are that the answer is not genetic in the traditional sense, and that sociocultural factors are highly implicated.

Ethnicity appears on the surface to be one of the major, if not the major, predictor of obesity risk in the United States. However, unraveling the concept of race/ethnicity further reveals that it is not a good predictor at all, because underneath lies the risk-focusing processes discussed earlier. The link between obesity and ethnicity is critical to thinking about culture-obesity connections, mainly because in the public health literature "ethnicity" and "culture" are often used interchangeably. That is, the literature assumes patterned behavioral differences between people categorized as African American and Mexican American, for example, that are cultural in origin and explain why obesity risk is shaped as it is. Further, public health often rolls out obesity as one of a long laundry list of "health disparities" from which minorities tend to suffer worst. The public health viewpoint poses substantial problems. Before addressing these directly, we need to examine the broad pattern of obesity risk by ethnicity.

Although the focus here is on variation in obesity risk by ethnicity/race in the United States, where the bulk of research using these variables has been applied, ethnic differences in obesity rates are commonly reported in other countries. For example, in New Zealand in 2006, the obesity rate for minority Maori was 41.7 percent, compared to 24.3 percent for Pakehas (European-ancestry New Zealanders) and 11 percent for Asians (New Zealand Ministry of Health 2008). Fiji, where I visit most summers, has major ethnic differences too, which while not well reported in the literature are instantly obvious to any visitor: indigenous Fijians (the majority), especially women, are at much more risk of obesity than are Indo-Fijians (Saito 1995).

How substantial is ethnic variation in obesity risk in the United States? Wang and Beydoun (2007) conducted a meta-analysis of nationally representative U.S. obesity data collected between 1990 and 2006, with a focus on the three most populous ethnic/race categories. The studies overall showed that people who categorized themselves as non-Hispanic Whites have lower risk of obesity at all ages than those self-classified as Black or Mexican American. Across all ages and genders, the prevalence of childhood obesity among African Americans, Mexican Americans, and Native Americans exceeds that of people who self-classified as belonging to other ethnic groups, including Asian and White. Major health surveys in the United States, such as NHANES, show not only that obesity in the United States has gone up during the last few years, but that women's rates are generally higher in minority than in majority race/ethnicity categories, sometimes very much so (see figure 4.5).

The most recent NHANES data analyses (1999–2004) show that Mexican American women are 1.3 times as likely, and Black women twice as likely, as White women to be overweight/obese. Among children and adolescents (two to nineteen years), Mexican American (but not African American) boys, especially in the age group six to eleven years, were more likely to be overweight/obese than White boys (1.7 times more likely for all ages). Among girls, Mexican American and African American girls were both around 1.5 times more likely to be overweight/obese than White girls, and this difference was statistically significant

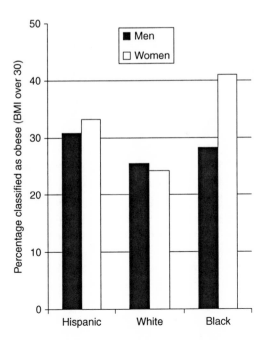

FIGURE 4.5 U.S. adult (twenty years old and up) obesity percentages by self-reported ethnicity, 2008. The data are age adjusted and based on self-reported height and weight rather than on direct anthropometric measures (see CDC 2008a).

(Ogden et al. 2006). In contrast, no racial or ethnic disparities were reported in male obesity rates; men who self-classified into one of the three main race/ethnicity categories (White, Mexican American, or Black) had no statistically significant difference in their risk of being overweight/obese. In 2008 National Health Examination Survey data, however, while White women still were less likely to be obese than were Black or Mexican American women, Black men were more likely to be obese than White men.

Local community- and school-based studies also have shown that Hispanic/Latino, native Hawaiian, Samoan, and American Indian children in the United States have for some considerable time (before the obesity epidemic) had a risk higher than that of non-Hispanic White children (Gordon-Larsen et al. 2003; Kumanyika 2007). These prevalence differences among children are related to a greater relative increase in prevalence among Mexican American and particularly non-Hispanic Black children during the past three decades, especially in children ages six and over (Freedman et al. 2006). Compared to the other major ethnic groups, African American children and youth have had the largest relative increase in obesity risk since the 1970s (Ogden et al. 2006). More recently, a much-elevated risk compared to whites has become evident among African American girls, especially over six years of age. These findings have led to the suggestion that relatively recent sociocultural and environmental changes (not fully specified or understood) may account for factors predisposing African American children to obesity compared to children in other minority groups (Kumanyika 1993). Of all the ethnic groups identified in the U.S. studies, Asian children's obesity rates tended to be the lowest.

Is the ethnic variation in risk that we observe in the United States, at least in children and women, related to genetic differences between those in each group? We know that, just as with gender, there are population differences in how fat distributes on the body, and these correlate with ethnicity classifications to some degree. African Americans are reported to have less visceral fat (associated with lower relative risk of obesity-related conditions such as diabetes and hypertension) than Whites or Hispanics of the same body weight (Bacha et al. 2003). Furthermore, in a range of studies that describe the metabolic profiles of various race/ethnicity categories, African Americans are reported to have lower rates of basal lipolysis (breakdown of fat stored in fat cells) than Whites (Danadian et al. 2001), and African American and Hispanics to have lower insulin sensitivity than whites at the same body size, meaning they are at risk for higher insulin resistance (Goran et al. 2002).

The significant scientific effort going into discovering and explaining the racial and ethnic bases of obesity risk, aimed at reducing health disparities in the United States, assumes that some critical population-based genetic factors are at play. At present this assumption is based mostly on "circumstantial evidence" (Caprio et al. 2008), because the exact relationship between race/ethnicity and comorbidities remains poorly defined. However, it is likely that in the larger picture genetic factors have nowhere near the explanatory power of variation in diet, exercise, lifestyle, and other factors shaped by culture and the social and physical contexts of lives. Thus, while genetic factors may well shape some part of the relationship between ethnicity and obesity, they are not the focus here. A recent consensus statement by the American Diabetes Association on the relationship between culture, ethnicity, race, and childhood obesity (Caprio et al. 2008) defines race and ethnicity as "social constructs" used to categorize populations on the basis of shared characteristics such as language or dietary preference. Furthermore, it notes, "race" categories account for only 3–7 percent of total human genetic diversity. In sum, there is conflicting evidence as to whether ethnicity independently predicts obesity risk in adults or children, once all other confounding factors such as income and socioeconomic status are taken into account (Lindquist, Reynolds, and Goran 1999; Wang 2001).

Building on the public health assumption of a causal link between ethnicity and obesity, we can observe a widespread and dominant assumption in weight-loss interventions that the most successful plans are those tailored to specific ethnic groups (Kumanyika 2008). A good example of the public health assumption that ethnicity predicts and explains most of the relevant cultural variation in obesity risk is represented in the consensus statement of the American Diabetes Association, Shaping America's Health, and the Obesity Society based on the conclusions of a seven-member panel of experts in endocrinology, nutrition, cardiology, gastroenterology, epidemiology, and anthropology. The statement provides a good overview of the current literature about variation in obesity-related behavior by ethnicity, and it uses a definition of culture not at odds with traditional anthropological definitions.

> Beliefs relating the normative and pragmatic rules for engaging in health-promoting behavior (diet and exercise) or leisure activity (watching television or playing video games) will change as individual members of an ethnic group experience and come to value innovative practices, while losing interest in and thereby disvaluing traditional practices. With both acculturation and globalization there are changes in preferences for certain foods and forms of leisure/physical activity, as well as educational and economic opportunities. These changes may differ by ethnic groups. For instance, first-generation Asian and Latino adolescents have been found to have higher fruit and vegetable consumption and lower soda consumption than whites. With succeeding generations, the intake of these items by Asians remains stable. In contrast, fruit and vegetable consumption by Latinos decreases while their soda consumption

increases, so that by the third generation their nutrition is poorer than that of whites. Acculturation to the U.S. is also significantly associated with lower frequency of physical activity participation in 7th-grade Latino and Asian American adolescents. . . . Culture is believed to contribute to disparities in childhood obesity in numerous ways. First, body image development occurs in a cultural context, and ethnic/cultural groups differ in their shared understandings as to valued and disvalued body image. For instance, perceived ideal body size for African American women is significantly larger than it is for white women, and African American men are more likely than non-Hispanic white men to express a preference for larger body size in women. The mean BMI at which white women typically express body dissatisfaction is significantly lower than that for African American women. . . . Given that women typically assume primary responsibility for the care, feeding, and education of children, including the transmission of shared cultural understandings, the beliefs that women possess with respect to their own body image have implications for their perception of and response to the body image of their children. This pattern may vary by ethnicity. For instance, non-Hispanic white mothers' dietary restraint or their perceptions of their daughters' risk of overweight can influence their young daughters' weight and dieting behaviors. In contrast, Latinas tend to prefer a thin figure for themselves but a plumper figure for their children. Culture influences child-feeding practices in terms of beliefs, values, and behaviors related to different foods. Affordability, availability of foods and ingredients, palatability, familiarity, and perceived healthfulness prompt immigrant families to retain or discard certain traditional foods and to adopt novel foods associated with the mainstream culture. Bilingual school-age children from immigrant Mexican households serve as agents of dietary acculturation by rejecting the lower-calorie traditional foods prepared at home and favoring the higher-calorie foods, beverages, and snacks they consume at school or see advertised on television and may resist efforts by their parents to restrict the availability of foods from the mainstream culture. . . . Cultural patterns of shared understandings influence food consumption in several ways. These shared understandings define which types of food are healthy and which are unhealthy. . . . Food is both an expression of cultural identity and a means of preserving family and community unity. While consumption of traditional food with family may lower the risk of obesity in some children (e.g., Asians), it may increase the risk of obesity in other children (e.g., African Americans). . . . Differences in levels and types of exposure to nutritional marketing may also account for cultural differences in patterns of nutrition. For instance, exposure to food-related television advertising was found to be

60% greater among African American children, with fast food as the most frequent category. Marketing strategies for food often target specific ethnic groups. This marketing, in turn, may produce alterations in belief systems as to the desirability of foods high in calories and low in nutrient density. . . . Culture influences preferences for and opportunities to engage in physical activity. As with nutrition, children model the types of physical activity undertaken by their parents; thus, a parent in a culture that views rest after a long workday as more healthy than exercise is less likely to have children who understand the importance of physical activity for health and well-being. Compared with their white counterparts, African American adolescents have greater declines in levels of physical activity with increasing age and are less likely to participate in organized sports. . . . Culture can influence the perception of risk associated with obesity. Studies of Latinos have found that many mothers of obese children believe their child to be healthy and are unconcerned about their child's weight, although these same parents are likely to believe that obese children in general should be taken to a nutritionist or physician for help with weight reduction. Among African American parents, there is greater awareness of acute health conditions than of obesity. . . . Culture can influence the utilization of health services, affecting the likelihood that childhood obesity can be prevented or effectively treated in specific ethnic groups. While ethnic differences in access to services can be attributed to differences in SES (e.g., higher proportions of Latinos lack health insurance or transportation to health care providers), several studies have pointed to differences in use of services even when access is available. Among Latino families, differences in patterns of service use have been found to be related to different beliefs about the cause, course, and cure of an illness, the stigma attached to particular illnesses, and interactions. (Caprio et al. 2008, 2570–2571)

This statement illustrates how ethnic categories are often used to mark patterned differences in how people choose to exercise and eat. Recent hypotheses regarding the elevated risk of obesity in Hispanics/Latinos suggest that such factors as lower physical activity levels and elevated caloric intake through sugary drinks are central (Crespo et al. 2001). Outside the cultural realm, alternative hypotheses for the elevated risk of obesity among Hispanic/Latinos include decreased metabolic utilization of fat due to undernutrition prior to migrating (Frisancho 2003). However, these hypotheses do not explain how "being Hispanic/Latino," for example, places people in the United States at elevated risk of being obese.

In this fairly standard view, culture is understood as having certain basic properties; shared rules for making sense of the world around us, learned and shaped by experience, enable us to behave in mutually interpretable ways. Some of the ways in which this view of culture is relevant to obesity include group members' view of fat bodies as beautiful, neutral, or ugly, and their views of obesity as a disease requiring medical treatment, a normal, nonmedical part of the human condition, or deserving of no notice at all.

Here we are distinguishing illness—the subjective experience of symptoms and suffering—from disease, a condition labeled by a medical practitioner (Kleinman 1988). The way we experience illness is intimately tied to the social systems in which we operate, as well as to the cultural factors that help us decide and label what has meaning for us, and what that meaning is. This is a well-worn and traditional view of culture that for the most part makes sense to anthropologists. It is useful, for example, to explain why the value of big bodies might vary from place to place and thus why in some contexts people would never consider trying to lose weight. But it is insufficient to explain much more, as we shall see once we talk about a systems approach to obesity. There is also growing recognition that culture is not monolithic, but that members of a society have quite different worldviews in some ways, even if they closely overlap in others.

In particular, ethnic categories do a poor job of capturing what can be substantial and important variations even in small-scale settings, although of course we would expect greater diversity in larger groups or more complicated social and ecological settings (such as modern cities or where there is diverse immigration). And we would expect some domains of knowledge (such as what foods constitute a good dinner) to be subject to more variation than others (such as what foods are suitable for fiestas). Also, men and women can understand how people relate to overweight based on quite different culturally derived conceptual frameworks, sometimes referred to as cultural models; the genders may therefore disagree on how much is too much food, what is good to eat, whether certain forms of exercise are desirable or appropriate, and what an ideal and acceptable body might look like.

The work of biocultural anthropologists William Dressler and Clarence Gravlee helps explain why it is helpful to think about ethnicity as not necessarily linked directly and monolithically to health outcomes like obesity, counter to some basic tendencies of the public health model. They note that in much of the public health literature, "ethnicity" refers indirectly to "culture" and both are conflated often with "race," at least in the United States. Dressler, Oths, and Gravlee (2005) provide "ethnoracial categories," culturally constructed or folk categories that denote essential differences in terms of biological ancestry. If we take this more critical approach, we can assume that "ethnicity" is at best a gloss, and more likely a mask, for the real and important relationships between culture and obesity. Based on the observation that ethnicity/race is the most commonly applied variable in U.S. public health research and often described as one of the major predictors of risk, the critical question arises. What are the underlying factors that explain why people placed in some racial/ethnic categories are at greater risk for obesity than those placed in other categories?

Obesity As an Index of Injustice

Reducing the risk of obesity among the most vulnerable groups in society requires that we develop tools and strategies for working with minority populations that do not explain behavioral variation with spurious theories of culture that equate an ethnic categorization with a worldview. We also need to think in more theoretically informed ways about how and why poverty, ethnicity, minority status, and so on coalesce to create obesity risk. Risk focusing and the human adaptability perspective provide one such strategy (see chapter 3). Environmental justice (EJ) provides another, one particularly useful for thinking about why ethnicity, minority status, income, occupation, SES, food access, place of residence, immigrant status, and who you know—each predictors of obesity risk within and across populations—tend to get tied together in complicated and often intractable ways to create risk. EJ explicates the relationships between social disadvantage and the distribution of amenities and disamenities in the physical (including the built) environment. Because it tends to focus on spatial relationships among these factors, EJ also provides a way to link variation on the ground to broader political-economic structures (in this case, discrimination in how cities are laid out).

Much EJ research to date has examined how disamenities, such as toxic dumps or air pollution, tend to be located in minority or lower-income neighborhoods, especially low-income, minority neighborhoods (Grineski, Bolin, and Boone 2007; Mennis and Jordan 2005; Morello-Frosch and Lopez 2006; Omer and Or 2005). This discriminatory distribution helps explain why minorities and the impoverished tend to be disproportionately burdened with negative health exposures. For example, a recent nationally representative analysis of physical activity facilities found that minority and low-income areas had worse facilities, and that this predicted lower levels of physical activity and higher obesity rates among adolescents in those areas (Gordon-Larsen et al. 2006). However, recognition is growing that the inequitable distribution of health-promoting environmental amenities in majority and wealthier areas—pleasant open spaces, clean air, and safe walking routes—may also contribute to health patterns (Pastor, Morello-Frosch, and Sadd 2005; Pellow and Brulle 2006).

Similar discriminatory patterns occur in some inner cities with regard to neighborhood access to healthy food sources. Lower-income and minority neighborhoods in the United States tend to be more likely to have food deserts and more fast-food outlets (Gallagher 2006; Horowitz et al. 2004; Morland, Diez Roux, and Wing 2002; Powell, Auld, et al. 2007; Sharkey and Horel 2008; Sloane et al. 2003). Areas around schools in and near minority and low-income neighborhoods may also have more fast-food advertising, placing residents in those areas at even greater risk of obesity. In sum, the risks of the built environment relevant to obesity are not evenly or fairly distributed by society, and assign further risk to the most vulnerable citizens. Amenity distribution becomes an even larger justice issue from an intergenerational perspective. However, the structure of the built environment and obesity prevalence are rarely considered in a justice framework (Rogge and Combs-Orme 2003), even though obesity in childhood may lead to lifelong social and physical health problems (Dietz 1997).

In an EJ approach, ethnicity in relation to health outcomes such as obesity is less related to being a member of a specific ethnic group and more a function of being a member of a minority. In the United States and many other places, being in a minority negatively impacts one's social and economic position and opportunity (one does not need to be in the numerical minority to be socially or economically disadvantaged by the broader political-economic system [Kumanyika 2007]). With this approach, it is possible to reframe the discussion about ethnicity and obesity and see that ethnic categories might be identifying not genetic differences or cultural differences but minority status and its accompanying social and political disadvantage (Dressler, Oths, and Gravlee 2005; Gravlee 2009; Kumanyika 2007). This is a very different way of thinking about culture in relation to obesity than anthropologists traditionally offer.

EJ and risk focusing are both conceptual models that provide theoretical rationales for why we would link certain factors across levels (for example, minority status, place of residence, and neighborhood built environments in the case of EJ, and socially based stigma and discrimination in the case of risk focusing). The models make good sense used in combination, with the former suggesting that location is critical and the latter emphasizing the importance of social (especially power) relations. Both suggest that ethnic categorization and discrimination reflect processes that tend to amplify the adverse environments with which people must cope, and to reduce the capacity to find socially or technologically based solutions.

People in obesogenic environments from the start are thus at increased risk of obesity. Where various systemic forms of oppression and discrimination exist (implicit in the EJ view), ethnicity/race is often bound with other sociocultural categories such as gender, class, and national origin. These systems of social inequality seldom act independently of one another, and interact on multiple levels to create a system of oppression at their intersection (an idea sometimes termed "intersectionality"; see, e.g., Collins 2000). It can be useful then to think about the effects of both gender and ethnicity variation on obesity risk as intertwined with each other and with the effects of SES, migrant status, urban-rural residence, and so on (Weber and Fore 2007).

Obesity and Social Networks

A different way to think about the social distribution of obesity is by analyzing an individual's social networks, that is, who individuals tend to associate with—webs of social connections among people who talk to each other, or the social relationships in which each of us is embedded in our everyday lives (Burt 1984; Valente 1995; Wellman 1979). A recent and much publicized study of a social network by Christakis and Fowler (2007) showed that, over time, individuals who had friends who became overweight/obese were more likely to become so as well, and obese people tended to increasingly cluster together. The effect of having friends who gained weight was greater with stronger friendships, greater for women than men, and greater for friendships of the same sex. The authors suggest that behind these findings might lie social norms, whereby "the fact that people are embedded in social networks and are influenced by the evident appearance and behaviors of those around them suggests that weight gain in one person might influence weight gain in others. Having obese social contacts might change a person's tolerance for being obese or might influence his or her adoption of specific behaviors (e.g., smoking, eating, and exercising)" (370).

As Christakis and Fowler present it, theirs is an individual-level argument for why people gain weight, not a social one, but there is the hint that a social argument might ultimately be more satisfying—that norms within our social group shape how we think about and act with our body. Obese people tend to report being most unhappy if they are around people who are not obese, as we will see here later.

A question we have been asking in our most recent work in low-income Latino neighborhoods in central Phoenix addresses such socially structured risk focusing: why do some people who live in the most obesogenic neighborhoods (unwalkable, unsafe food deserts) nonetheless maintain excellent nutritional health and healthy body sizes? We suspect the answer is cultural and social, including cultural rules about sharing and reciprocity, such as helping each other access food and transportation through social networks, and social network analysis (Burt 1984; Wellman 1979) is a way to link variability in the complex social contexts of people's everyday lives with their ability to cope with poor food environments. Social networks in our Phoenix research are a conduit for sharing not only food, but also food-relevant knowledge and norms. While little research at present systematically links social networks with variation in dietary outcomes at the household level (for one exception, see Wutich and McCarty 2008), it is reasonable to assume that risk buffering might result from sharing food or food stamps, nutritional advice, and guidance; granting small loans; and pooling food buying and transportation (see, e.g., Sherraden and Barrera 1996). Network norms and configurations may also stabilize food supplies during cyclical shortages (Lomnitz 1977), particularly for children.

Social network analysis may be particularly germane in Latino communities, because systems of reciprocal exchange, including large kin networks with high rates of interaction and visitation, are important within traditional Mexican society and remain important to many migrants in the United States (Kana'iaupuni et al. 2005; Keefe 1984). Amber Wutich's work in Mexico (Wutich and McCarty 2008) and our own work in South Phoenix (Szkupinski Quiroga, Brewis, and Wutich 2008) suggest that Latino families with the strongest local, kin-based social networks may do more pooling of purchasing and are more likely to eat at home. Similarly, those more tied into the local Latino community may have access to healthy, cheap, home-prepared meals that are sold at others' kitchen tables.

Because not all ties within networks are supportive, social networks can create—as much as solve—the problems of living in a low-resource setting (Menjivar 2000). Being obliged to follow group rules for preparing or sharing food in a household, for example, can impose difficult challenges and commitments. In our South Phoenix work, we suspect that some network structures or types of ties promote or encourage better nutrition, while others promote resistance to positive nutritional change. The idea of risk focusing also helps us think about how the buffering effects that culture can provide might become strained and worn thin under poverty conditions (Schell 1997, 76); the more stratified a society is, the more likely this is to happen. For example, if we follow the social network argument, under conditions of severe social and resource stress (conditions common in many communities with the current economic downturn), social obligations to share with others might be damaging as easily as they could be supportive—an issue we are testing in South Phoenix using a household-based study.

Modeling Complex and Dynamic Biocultural Causation

In this chapter we have seen results of epidemiological studies that represent the cornerstone of the public health approach; they emphasize how exposure to various stressors shapes the pattern of ill health at the population level. You are at elevated risk for obesity if you are poor, female, a minority, or an American (or Nauruan); if you live in the suburbs; or if you have overweight or obese friends. Of course obesity is a complex, multifactorial condition influenced by interconnected social, cultural, physiological, environmental, developmental, and genetic factors. Moreover, obesity is not a constant: it is possible for people to go from slim to fat, or fat to slim. At a slightly higher scale of consideration, structural inequities that allocate amenities differently across and within communities contribute to obesity distributions.

Distal or ultimate (or upstream) explanations for the obesity epidemic include those linked to food policies. At the national and city levels, the post–World War II rise of suburban living and dependence on cars for transportation is associated with an increase in obesity, while at the community or neighborhood level, low walkability and poor food environments contribute. At the family, social network, or household level, norms related to food or exercise may shape risk, and at the individual level, individual choices about food and exercise are important. Finally, at the molecular and organ levels, we can think about individual as well as population variation in the propensity to convert carbohydrates to fat.

At the individual level, a range of proximate (or downstream) explanations of why people are overweight mostly come down to people taking in more calories than they exercise off. Viewed at other levels, obesity is simultaneously an expression of structural inequities, a disease of poverty, and a result of neighborhood shaping of individual dietary and exercise options. The way in which obesity is explained depends completely on the scalar level at which one addresses it.

Figure 4.6 provides a visual graphic of various levels that can help us understand how obesity risk is shaped, from genetic disposition "under the skin" to macropolitical forces at the global level. The assignment of items across these levels is somewhat arbitrary, for example, are social networks above family and at the level of local institutions, are they at the level of family, or do they link the two? At which level is learning about food? Where does ethnicity fit into all this? But this framework gives us a way to start thinking about how multiple factors might explain quite different individual pathways to obesity. It may be useful to conceptualize obesity as a body form that emerges at the interface of many interacting levels of causative explanation. An advantage of this type of model is that it recognizes that obesogenic environments interact with biological dispositions to shape obesity risk.

One of the large challenges facing obesity research generally is the limited usefulness of traditional statistics for getting at the interconnections between the possible explanations and levels of explanations that shape obesity risk in more than a very preliminary way. Current methods in biomedical research cannot account for more than three levels of behavioral or biological influences at the same time, and existing hierarchical models find it difficult to nest the study of individuals in any context beyond families and schools. Likewise, little consideration has been given to the multiple levels of biological data and the integration of these with environmental factors.

On the one hand, traditional epidemiological approaches, which are what many of the studies discussed so far have applied, do a good job of describing the general pattern of obesity risk but a relatively poor job of moving beyond individual risk factors to the larger cumulative social, cultural, and ecological processes that explain that more proximate variation in risk (Krieger 1994). Epidemiology focuses to the exclusion of almost all else on a model of disease,

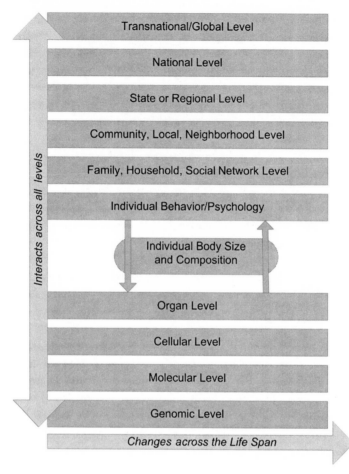

FIGURE 4.6 A conceptual model of levels and related domains that shape obesity risk.
Adapted from NIH 2008.

and one in which the hosts of the disease (individuals) interact with disease
agents (high-fat food) in specified physical environments (inner-city neighborhoods) (see Oakes 2008). The model excludes other people and any of their
collective emergent social or economic phenomena—norms, culture, social
organization, and policy (Oakes 2008; Trostle 2005; Worthman and Kohrt 2005).

On the other hand, many of the ultimate explanations of obesity, such as
the commodification/globalization explanations that opened chapter 1, invoke
macroscale political-economic arguments that—while based on an interpretation of the epidemiological evidence—remain uncoupled with and untested
against the dynamic processes that must underlie them. That is, they do not
empirically link back down to what people are eating and drinking except in an
indirect way. In recent years, the more common way of analyzing health (including

obesity) data to understand causal effects has been regression-based or multilevel analysis. Multilevel models are an extension of fairly standard regression models that look at how differences in exposures of various kinds lead to individual variation in weight. These approaches necessarily simplify what are most certainly complex processes, and theorize most of these as unidirectional.

Obesity research (and health research more generally) needs analytical tools that can simultaneously and empirically (quantitatively) test the causal paths and feedback loops among proximate and distal, biological, environmental, and cultural drivers of what people eat and how they move as they shape risk. Newer methods such as agent-based modeling hold great promise for addressing these challenges, as they allow us to ask how alterations at a much wider range of levels might shape the phenomena with which we are proximally concerned (Anderson 1999; Auchincloss and Diez Roux 2008). To understand such questions as why certain groups are at elevated risk or why obesity is increasing or leveling out, we need think beyond causal chains to causal loops (Newell et al. 2007). One of the useful things that agent-based models allow is consideration of tipping points. For example, as you gain weight, there may be a tipping point at which you become cast as overweight when social and economic opportunities start to collapse, reshaping your social environment so you are more likely to be around more overweight people and thus be less motivated to lose weight.

In this chapter, we have started to think about a variety of ways in which the concept of culture can be applied in obesity research, at different levels and using some quite different approaches. In the next chapters, we look more explicitly and purposefully about what we mean by culture in relation to obesity, and especially how we can study it.

5

Culture and Body Ideals

Ultimately, our bodies represent cultural facts, just as they do biological ones. Body size is imbued with cultural meaning in all human societies, perhaps because it is such an obvious physical trait. The definition of what constitutes an ideal, attractive, or acceptable body is, especially viewed in historical perspective, one of the most highly ecologically and culturally varied aspects of female attractiveness (Brown and Konner 1987; Sobal and Stunkard 1989). Though seemingly highly flexible and potentially variable among groups, cultural values about attractive bodies tend to be strongly, consistently, and widely held within groups.

Yet like many things that are innately cultural, we take for granted our understanding of which bodies are too big, too small, or just right. Growing up in New Zealand, I never gave my body size much thought. I would have described myself as normal and acceptable—just a good healthy Kiwi girl with the requisite meat on her bones. But when I moved to the United States in my early twenties, it dawned on me that I was perhaps a little chunky. When I was living in Micronesia a couple of years later, people told me I was far too skinny; friends pushed food at me, genuinely concerned that if I did not plump up, I would have trouble getting a husband. My body measured exactly the same in all three places, but people's reactions to it were utterly different, and these made a profound difference to how I experienced and understood my own body on a day-to-day basis.

Understanding how people differently understand body size within and across human societies is critical to thinking through the global problem of obesity because it is possible to argue that the major costs that accrue to most people with big, fat bodies are social rather than physical. By social costs, I mean the manifestations of the profound stigma attached to fat, such as blocked opportunities, social rejection, low self-esteem, and the loss of social agency and

power. In many industrialized societies, especially as education and socioeconomic status increase, obesity is understood culturally not only as a harbinger
of disease and ill health but also as morally bad and thus socially discrediting of
the individual. The negative cultural values regarding big bodies are so profound, oft communicated, and pervasive in contemporary Western society
(especially for women) that they are somewhat taken for granted. We collectively as a society *know* that fat bodies are unhealthy (even though, as we have
seen, the science is equivocal), and we may emotionally relate to the finding
that many Americans say they would rather be divorced, die younger, or be
blind than be obese (Schwartz et al. 2006).

However, this view of big and especially fat bodies as unhealthy, shameful,
and bad is historically recent, and certainly not culturally universal. As recently
as the 1980s, the view of fatness as disease or illness was still sufficiently a
berrant in the cross-cultural record to be labeled by some anthropologists a
culture-bound syndrome (Ritenbaugh 1982). Despite the significant global
spread of the thinness ideal over the last two decades, a range of societies still
fundamentally views big, fat bodies as morally good, as well as healthy and
attractive. The contrast of this perspective to what we observe in the West offers
an opportunity to rethink our cultural embrace of the idea that fat bodies are
bad, unhealthy, and ugly.

But many (though not all) historically fat-tolerant or fat-positive societies
are increasingly expressing thinner body ideals, even as their populations grow
in girth. Thin idealism seems to follow television and other culturally powerful
influences through media penetration. If negative ideas about fat bodies are
spreading globally, and especially if the stigma attached to these ideas accom-
panies the spread, then the social as well as physical costs of weight gain globally could be profound in the years ahead, and obesity could influence people's
social lives in completely new ways.

This chapter and the next lay out the core published evidence on variation
in how people understand big bodies, and a range of approaches to studying
and interpreting that variability, including some theoretical approaches that
apply fundamentally different definitions of culture, which naturally lead to
sometimes contradictory and irreconcilable conclusions and recommenda-
tions; the ultimate result is a richer set of understandings.

One further note: almost every aspect of how body weight is understood,
classified, and responded to in social contexts differs for men versus women. In
the West, weight experiences and gender are so tightly enmeshed as to be fundamentally inseparable (Bordo 1993). While, as discussed earlier, women are more
likely on average to be obese, they are less likely (as we will see in this chapter)
to be satisfied with their bodies, less likely to judge them accurately, more likely
to suffer from stigma attached to obesity, and more likely to be dieting or to be
diagnosed with eating disorders. There is more written about women and bodies

from a cultural perspective, and the social ante is much higher. For all of these reasons, in this chapter, as in my own work, I focus on women's bodies more than on men's.

Body Image and Body Ideals

The "very thin" ideal for women in the West became the norm only after the 1950s (Walden 1985), although size consciousness had been evident for a century. The Human Relations Area File (HRAF) is a standardized database that contains information on cultural norms from a wide range of societies, collected by anthropologists doing long-term ethnographic studies over the last century. Of 325 listed societies, there are comments about female body ideals for 38. Of those, just 7 were noted by an ethnographer to prefer thin or to abhor fat; the remaining 31 prefer plump to thin. These plump-preferring societies are found in all regions of the world historically, except for Asia (Brown and Konner 1987). Notably, however, there is no record in the HRAF of a society that prefers extreme (morbidly) obese bodies. The cross-cultural evidence of preference for largeness in men's bodies in the HRAF is spottier: of the twelve societies for which an ethnographer made specific notes about cultural preferences, each preferred tall, muscular men. What the HRAF data suggest in totality is that when body size is viewed across human societies, a preponderance of groups traditionally prefer plump bodies on women and many have no concept of excess fat (obesity) as a bad thing (Brown and Konner 1987).

One of the easiest ways to conceptualize and test hypotheses about cross-cultural variation in people's conceptions of large bodies is through the comparative study of body image (see appendix C for an explanation of body image scales). Body image refers to the way people perceive their body size and shape, and how their estimates compare to their actual size. In the majority of body image studies, thin preference has been evident. That is, women in particular pick a slim ideal as the body they would prefer, and this slim body is smaller on average than both the size they are and the size they perceive themselves to be. However, it is important to recognize that body image studies mainly come out of psychology, and overwhelmingly they have been concerned with body image in the United States and other industrial countries (such as Australia, the United Kingdom, European nations, and New Zealand), and that by far the greatest number of studies have been conducted with female undergraduates (an ever-ready research population). From the perspective of the cross-cultural record, these findings provide a limited picture of the total possible range of human variability. Nonetheless, in the last fifteen years more studies have been conducted in a wider range of societies, on older, less educated sample populations, and with men. These new data help give a better picture of body ideals globally.

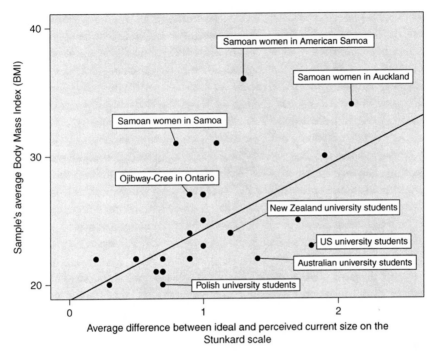

FIGURE 5.1 A cross-cultural comparison of average differences between women's ideal and perceived size, drawing on data from the studies listed in appendix C, table I. On average, women in every culture reported wanting to be smaller than their perceived size.

In figure 5.1, I have pooled the results of all the body image studies I could locate that used the same scale, in this case the nine-figure Figural Rating Scale developed by Stunkard and his colleagues (Stunkard, Sorensen, and Schulsinger 1983) or its adaptations (e.g., Fallon and Rozin 1985). This data set allows a good comparison of studies across quite different cultural contexts—Native American, Middle Eastern, Asian-Pacific, and Eastern European populations, as well as those of the major industrialized nations; the list of studies and their primary findings appears in appendix C. The results in figure 5.1 include only studies where average BMI measures were available for each sample. I have not included clinical samples, such as people with conditions such as anorexia or bulimia, who tend to have much slimmer ideals than are reported in these community-based samples. As is the case with many psychometric tools, the majority of the data in the literature is drawn from samples of university (especially psychology) students. Studies across a range of cultural settings are relatively few, but pulled together they allow us to make some general observations about the cross-cultural trends.

The most obvious observation, upon looking at figure 5.1 and the data in appendix C, is that in every study reported using the Figural Rating Scale, women on average report they want to be smaller than the size they think they are. This finding shows clearly that, at least in the populations sampled, while there are differences in what people think of as the ideal body, a thin ideal (around 2.8–3 on the Stunkard scale) tends to be the average in most places, with a mean rating of 4 on the Stunkard scale the very highest value observed. A second observation is that the higher BMI groups tend to show a greater disparity between the size they think they are and size they would like to be; that is, higher BMI samples do not necessarily have larger ideal bodies, but a greater gap between the size they identify as ideal and the size they think they are. The Samoan data are a case in point, reflecting a very slim ideal even though the women have some of the higher average BMIs of the groups sampled. The third primary conclusion we can draw from these studies is that not only Anglo samples but also many others—especially those of similarly educated, younger people in other countries—tend to report lower ideal body sizes on average than other groups.

Comparative studies using other body image tools have shown similar cross-cultural variation. Ugandan undergraduates view larger bodies more positively than do matched same-age British undergraduates (Furnham and Baguma 1994), as do women in Samoa when compared to age-matched Sydney women (Wilkinson, Ben-Tovim, and Walker 1994). Israeli women prefer a larger body as their ideal compared to U.S. women of the same age (Barak et al. 1994), and the discrepancy between ideal and estimated body size is smaller for Arab undergraduate women than for undergraduate Americans (Ford, Dolan, and Evans 1990). Caribbean (Simeon et al. 2003) and Tongan (Craig et al. 1999) women have been reported as having more positive attitudes toward large body sizes than Anglo women have. In our research, it has been clear that Samoans are unlikely to regard themselves as overweight or obese even when they are very large, and even if they identify a slim ideal, large Samoans are no more motivated to become slim than are their smaller-bodied peers, a pattern also seen in other Pacific Island groups (Brewis et al. 1998).

Another study contrasted Sámi (formerly termed "Laplanders"), a coastal fishing, trapping, and reindeer and sheepherding group indigenous to northern Scandinavia, to Finns in Helsinki and to Britons. There were striking differences in how the groups responded to higher BMI figures, with Sámi preferring much larger figures up to BMIs of 35, for example, as well as less curvy (more boxy) figure shapes than the other groups (Swami and Tovée 2007).

In another study, Tovée and colleagues (2006) recruited three groups of participants from South Africa—ethnic Zulus, Zulu migrants to London, and Anglo Londoners—to rate grey-scale frontal photographs of women of known BMI for health and attractiveness. The Anglo Londoners rated low- and high-BMI pictures the least attractive and least healthy (an inverted-U-shaped distribution). By comparison, both Zulu groups rated much higher BMIs attractive and healthy and gave high attractiveness ratings to pictures with high BMI. Peak attractiveness BMI (the picture that the most people responded positively to) was 20 for Londoners, 26.5 for Zulus, and 24 for migrant Zulus. Zulus chose a peak BMI of 30 when asked to rate the healthiness of body shapes, compared to 21 for Anglos and 25 for the Zulu migrants (Tovée et al. 2006). In a similarly designed study, men in Kuala Lumpur and London showed a preference for figures with a BMI of about 20, while those in Malaysia preferred a BMI of about 25 (Swami and Tovée 2005).

Preference for larger body sizes was also evident in a study of 249 Sahraoui (Moors) living in Laayoun, a city in the south of Morocco, 80 percent of whom were overweight or obese based on BMI measures. Using a 1–9 figure-rating scale (not the Stunkard FRS scale), the women selected a heavier ideal image for themselves (mean 4.9) than the smaller size they rated as healthy (mean of 4.3). Over 80 percent of the women reported that they had tried to gain weight at some time, and most felt their weight was appropriate. Of the fifty women who did want to change their weight, forty-two were trying to gain rather than lose weight (Rguibi and Belahsen 2006).

Besides a large body of evidence for cross-national differences in preferred and acceptable body size, ethnicity predicts marked differences within countries in how people judge different body sizes. For example, Anglo Americans have a slimmer ideal or less positive view of large bodies than have Mexican Americans, African Americans, Puerto Rican Americans, and sometimes Asian Americans (Greenberg and LaPorte 1996; Massara 1979; Parker et al. 1995; Streigel-Moore et al. 1995). Studies show that in the United States, African American women report larger body ideals, and are also reported as much more satisfied with their bodies, than their White counterparts (e.g., Rucker and Cash 1992). They are also less likely to diet, and more likely to either correctly estimate or underestimate their weight (Desmond et al. 1989; Williamson et al. 2000), even though they are heavier on average than U.S. White women. A meta-analysis of fifty-five studies examining differences in body satisfaction found that white women were much less satisfied with their bodies than were African American women (Roberts et al. 2006).

In terms of response to obesity, Latinas are more likely than U.S. Anglo women to rate themselves attractive, even at higher weights (Altabe 1998). The results of studies with Asian respondents have found equivocal or confusing results—in some cases Asian women are less likely than Anglo women to express body satisfaction, and in other cases they express more satisfaction. Still other studies show that they are similar to White women in their responses regarding body satisfaction and weight concern, or that their fear of fat is even more pronounced (Akan and Grilo 1995; Cachelin et al. 2002; Mintz and Kashubeck 1999; Sanders and Heiss 1998; Tsai, Hoerr, and Song 1998). In contrast, the studies looking at ethnic variation in body image or body satisfaction among men, at least in the United States, mostly found no significant variation (Cachelin et al. 2002; Mintz and Kashubeck 1999).

There is a basic question about whether the differences seen across ethnic groups in the United States are cultural differences specifically related to ethnicity or reflective of variation in other aspects of socioecology, such as the proportion of their social network that are overweight, SES, education, and the like. (This is similar to the debate discussed in chapter 4 about whether variation in obesity rates is a result of ethnicity or covariants.) We could expect, for example, that in subgroups where obesity is more common (such as in low-income, minority neighborhoods), there might be larger body norms and more body satisfaction, simply because people are interacting more often with larger-sized individuals. At present we not have no good evidence one way or the other; as noted in chapter 4, people tend to get fatter as their friends get fatter, which certainly makes this an interesting proposition to test. In regard to SES, there is good evidence that thinner ideals tend to be associated with increased wealth. For example, controlling for ethnicity, Swami and Tovée (2005, 2007) report that low-SES observers tend to prefer a higher BMI in a potential partner than do high-SES observers. Some small studies have controlled for body size, age, and ethnicity in their analyses and have found that African American and Latino men and women overall still reported greater body satisfaction and less overestimation of weight than did White men and women (Smith et al. 1999), and other studies have found that the effects of ethnicity disappear once these other factors are controlled for (Caldwell, Brownell, and Wilfley 1997).

Cachelin and colleagues found that, once SES and age were controlled for, there was no real difference between Hispanic, White, and Black women in their ideal body size and in the body sizes they selected as most attractive and acceptable. One way to interpret this finding is that the cultural differences are minor compared to such factors as BMI and SES, which might be much more powerful determinants of body-size perceptions and preferences (Cachelin et al. 2002). Alternatively, there is some debate in the psychological literature about whether the higher body satisfaction reported among African American women is due to different perceptions of ideal and acceptable bodies or to higher overall self-esteem (Cachelin et al. 2002; Haile and Johnson 1989; Henriques and Calhoun 1999; Roberts et al. 2006), since low self-esteem predicts greater body distortion.

A third possibility is that as studies increasingly recognize that racial/ethnic categories encompass or even obscure very culturally diverse groups, and as they accordingly assign culturally more meaningful analysis categories, we will achieve more satisfying and meaningful results. For example, the ambiguous results regarding Asians in the United States are probably at least partially explained by the profound cultural diversity of the category. For example, South Indians from rural Bangladesh and Japanese from Tokyo (and hence migrants from both these groups in the United States) might react very differently to body image scales.

In slim-preferring sample populations, regardless of their place of origin, it is also widely reported that women not only tend to pick a body ideal for themselves that is significantly smaller than their perceived body size, but also often fail to accurately identify their actual body size (often overestimating it on the body image scales). Furthermore, they are also often inaccurate in predicting what men think is the most attractive body size. This body distortion pattern was first observed in publication in 1985, when Fallon and Rozin demonstrated that U.S. undergraduate women could not accurately predict the body shape their male peers found most attractive, instead selecting a much slimmer figure. In comparison, men on average more accurately predicted women's ideals and chose an ideal size that reflected their relative satisfaction with their own body (Fallon and Rozin 1985).

This pattern of women's distorted perception of the body found most attractive by the other gender has been replicated with other samples of undergraduate women, parents of students, partners, and adolescents and older women in the United States and other industrialized nations (Cohn and Adler 1992; Cohn et al. 1987; Furnham and Radley 1989; Huon, Morris, and Brown 1990; Lamb et al. 1993; Rozin and Fallon 1988; cf. Furnham, Hester, and Weir 1990). In fact, body image distortion (the inability to correctly identify one's body size, especially to overestimate it) is so common among young women in industrialized nations that it can be considered a normative part of their psychologies, along with the high levels of body dissatisfaction that accompany it (Rodin, Silberstein, and Striegel-Moore 1985). In the West at least, psychology research has shown that body distortion and body dissatisfaction are correlated with risk for excessive levels of behaviors designed to attain and maintain (extreme) slimness, including restrained eating and refusal to eat (anorexia), induced vomiting, overexercising, and drug use for appetite suppression (Walsh and Devlin 1998).

Until recently, when compared to women, men in most studied industrialized countries have tended to be more satisfied with their bodies and able to more accurately estimate their body sizes on body image scales (see, e.g., Kostanski, Fisher, and Gullone 2004). While overweight men increasingly report a desire to be slimmer, this ideal has not reached the level of body distortion observed in women. Furthermore, men are much more likely to report themselves as underweight and much more likely than women to report they want to be larger (albeit due to an increase in muscle rather than fat). A number of studies have suggested that the major reason for women's body distortion is their exposure to Western media images of ultraslim women, which, internalized, results in distorted self-images and conceptions of other's judgments of their bodies (e.g., Martin and Gentry 1997; Ogden and Mundray 1996; Shaw and

Waller 1995). This pattern of female (and increasingly male) body distortion does not tend to occur in societies where women report larger body ideals and greater body satisfaction, nor does media exposure in and of itself predict body dissatisfaction.

The Ecology of Body Image

How is body image transforming in a globalizing world where ecological and social change often occurs apace with the spread of television, movies, and mass marketing? The few cross-sectional studies of how body image varies for migrants from less developed countries who move to industrial urban centers compared to nonmigrants suggest that as people from more fat-tolerant societies move into fat-abhorrent ones, their body ideals can shrink. Several studies of Asian British and Asian American women have shown that their body ideals can exceed even mainstream Anglo ideals of thinness, even though they have smaller mean body sizes than Anglos (Wardle et al. 1993). Scott and colleagues (2007) compared a small sample of Bangladeshi migrants in London to nonmigrants in northeast Bangladesh and found that compared to nonmigrant men, migrant men showed a preference for leaner women's bodies. However, earlier cross-cultural studies, such as one showing that Kenyan migrants to Britain report body ideals similar to in situ Kenyans and larger than those of other British residents (Furnham and Alibhai 1983), indicate this may be a relatively recent phenomenon.

The study Stephen McGarvey and I conducted with Samoans in the mid-1990s, already mentioned, found that downward shifts in idealized body size may be more pronounced among Samoan migrants moving into ecologically modern settings (Auckland) than in settings where increasing exposure to ecological/economic modernization has been more gradual (American Samoa and Samoa). Moreover, new ideas about the positive value of smaller bodies have been acquired less rapidly by Samoans in American Samoa and Samoa than in the Auckland Samoan population. According to ethnographic studies and historical records, larger bodies represent chiefly status, power (*mana*), and affluence; obesity is considered the product of an individual's high status (Gould 1994; Howard 1986). Aside from the chiefly classes, premodern Samoan bodies were tall and well built, but not characteristically obese (Sullivan 1921; Wilkes 1856).

As part of our study, we also conducted a series of interviews with Samoan men and women and collected body image ratings and anthropometric measures. The study, which included 65 Samoans in Auckland, New Zealand (see Brewis et al. 1998), and was carried out in conjunction with the Ola Fa'autauta project (Swinburn, Amosa, and Bell 1997); we also recruited 160 respondents from eight villages in urban and rural Samoa and 76 people from the urban center of Pago

Pago, American Samoa, in conjunction with the Brown University Adiposity and Cardiovascular Disease Risk Study (Chin-Hong and McGarvey 1996). The American Samoan segment of the research was conducted only with women; the other samples comprise both genders. Also, in Samoa and American Samoa, Samoans dominate numerically, socially, and economically. In Auckland, Samoans are a minority immigrant group (first and second generation) within a dominant Pakeha (white European) cultural milieu, where exposure to thin-depicting media is also considerably greater than in Samoa and American Samoa.

Each participant in the study was asked to locate on the adapted Stunkard 9-point body image scale (see p. 156) their perceptions of their own current size, size they would most like to be, average and ideal size for their age group, most attractive size, and upper and lower limits of acceptable body size in a mate. On the scale of opposite-gender bodies, participants identified the body size they found most attractive, average and ideal size for their age group, and upper and lower limits of acceptable body size in a mate.

One intent in the design of this study was to compare across sites how Samoan body image and body size were transforming in relation to each other and to various socioecological factors (such as entry into the cash economy) as Samoans increasingly engaged with the process of modernization. Studies that define modernization solely on the basis of location like this can mask a variety of lifeways that represent different levels of modernization for individuals (Bindon and Baker 1985), so we also looked at the relationship between body image and individual measures of modernization such as participant's occupation, education, and material possessions. Examples of traditional occupations are farmer, chief, or housewife, while nontraditional occupations include teacher or engineer.

Our study showed that Samoan men and women, even those in the much more traditional setting of rural Samoa, identified ideal body sizes significantly smaller than the sizes they perceived themselves to be on average (table 5.1). This is an interesting finding given that Samoa has for some time been considered one of the societies that culturally values large bodies. While a cross-sectional design such as we used cannot determine the causal relationships between decreasing body image, increasing body size, and ecological modernization, we offer the following suggestions about this complex relationship as the most reasonable interpretation of the results.

First, with increasing modernization, women acquire slimmer body ideals. The slimmest ideals occur in the most modern site, Auckland, while women in Samoa select larger ideals on average. When compared, the Samoa and Auckland data suggest that Samoan body ideals are becoming smaller as modernization progresses, despite significant increases in actual body size. Second, slim body ideals can be acquired in the absence of the profound changes in body size that are associated (albeit indirectly) with the caloric enrichment of ecological modernization.

Women in Samoa (the least modern environment) picked an ideal body size significantly smaller than their perceived current size, just as women did in the more modern setting of Auckland. Third, although the Samoans sampled are acquiring the idea of slim fashion, this acquisition is less rapid or less salient in environments where Samoans remain the dominant cultural group.

Finally, there are gender differences in the speed, salience, or both of acquiring slim ideals during the process of modernization, which is notable but not surprising. While men in both Samoa and Auckland identified body ideals significantly smaller than their perceived current size, men in the more modern setting (Auckland) selected an ideal size that was larger and closer to their current perceived body weight than did men in Samoa. This gender difference in body image, where male ideals tend to be less extreme than female, is now conventional wisdom in studies of body image in Western populations (Fallon and Rozin 1985; Furnham, Hester, and Weir 1990).

The results of our study show that of the three groups, American Samoans, who have bigger bodies and live in a social setting where Samoans remain dominant socially, are maintaining more achievable ideal values. Another

TABLE 5.1

Samoan Body Image by Gender at Three Sites, 1994–1996

	Women			Men	
	Aukland	American Samoa	Samoa	Aukland	Samoa
Mean BMI	34.1 (7.9, 22–59)	35.7 (7.7, 20–64)	30.5 (5.8, 19–47)	33.5 (6.8, 21–49)	28.9 (5.3, 18–40)
% obese (> BMI 32)	55.0	64.9	36.3	66.6	27.9
Mean estimate of current size from scale	45.2 (24.6)	48.9 (16.6)	36.5 (13.7)	53.9 (20.9)	37.2 (12.1)
Mean ideal body size from scale	23.8 (10.7)	35.1 (11.9)	29.1 (10.5)	39.5 (5.8)	28.4 (9.0)
Mean disparity (%) between perceived current and ideal body size	48.5 (17.1)	37.6 (17.1)	39.2 (17.6)	35.1 (17.2)	39.9 (14.1)
% content with current size	7.5	19.3	45.8	16.6	32.5

Note: Standard deviations and ranges are given in parentheses.

important finding was that although women in the more traditional setting of Samoa might identify a thin ideal, the thin ideal itself had much less salience for them than for women in the other two groups. That is, many more reported they were happy with their current body size, they felt no related need to lose weight, and they were not dieting or exercising to reach their ideal size. Samoans in all three sites accurately predicted the size the opposite gender finds attractive, both in general and in their own age groups. Further, men and women accurately predicted the average size of bodies in their age groups as perceived by both genders. This finding is quite different from that of studies in the United States, most of which were conducted with psychology undergraduates.

To address the proposition that media exposure might be driving the pattern of body size misestimation, we can compare Samoan women and men in more media-exposed Auckland to those in less media-exposed Samoa. Both groups were equally accurate in their assessments of their peers' attractive body preferences, which suggests that the media model is insufficient to explain population variation in women's ability to estimate men's ideals of women's bodies. An important distinction that may explain this different result in Samoa is that body form is a much less important vehicle for social, economic, conjugal, or reproductive success for Samoan women than it is for female undergraduates in the United States, for example. Moreover, in relatively collectivistic Samoan society, attractiveness has less salience in marriage decisions than do status and family, vital social themes and thus important considerations. The same holds true in nearby Fiji (Becker 1995, 2004).

Economic and ecological change, as part of the process of modernization and globalization, might promote changes in body preferences, as the few studies of this issue suggest, although the specific mechanisms that underlie this cultural shift are not well understood. Changes in body preferences might follow exposure to media images, such as when television is introduced, which explains part of the change in Fiji (as we will see in chapter 6), or might not, as we have found in Samoa. Or the body preference changes could be linked in part to the emergence of fat bodies in areas previously dominated by thin ones.

Generally, it appears that ideal or desired body sizes often decrease markedly with increasing exposure to contemporary Western notions of slimness and to economic modernity, and shrink even further in industrial settings as socioeconomic status increases (Goldblatt, Moore, and Stunkard 1965). However, there is no simple pattern in the change in body ideals with modernization or globalization, and the relationship between slimming body ideals and degree of modernization is not necessarily linear. Raphael and Lacey (1992) have proposed that the negative effects of acculturation on body image are more dramatic—that is, they occur more rapidly and notably—when cultural contact and assimilation are forced (such as during processes like migration) than when a society gradually acquires new values from external sources. While some studies support this proposition, others do not. Akan and Grilo (1995) show that degree of assimilation with mainstream U.S. culture appears unrelated to ethnic differences in body image in some groups.

We are still far from understanding in a fundamental sense how, when, or why these transformations in views about bodies occur in the context of economic modernization, arguably one of the most powerful aspects of contemporary ecological change. Further, despite the changes in body size that occur during the process of modernization, how apparent changes in body image articulate with actual changes in body size remains unclear. The caloric enrichment of modernization almost always promotes a trend to larger bodies (McGarvey et al. 1989) that is counter to apparent downward trends in notions of ideal body size. Thus, slim idealism seems to be one particular and powerful idea that has spread with modernization, as the Samoan case makes evident. The reasons that slim ideals are accepted or resisted and how salient the ideals become, however, is much more complicated than simply exposure to Western media. What we do know is that the change is generally one-sided—toward the dominant Western norm of thin idealism/fat aversion, rather than toward fat-neutral or fat-positive values.

Body Shape Preferences

A number of studies have looked for systematic patterns to people's responses to differently shaped bodies cross-culturally, especially by comparing waist-to-hip ratio (WHR) preferences. WHR is calculated by dividing waist circumference by hip circumference. A low WHR describes a more curvaceous (hourglass) figure, and a high WHR indicates a more apple-shaped one. Evolutionary psychologist Devendra Singh has done a series of studies describing men's preferences for specific body shapes as an evolved aspect of their mating strategies, by comparing how samples of men in various societies respond to differing WHR in women. A female WHR of 0.7 has been selected as the most attractive by men in myriad Western samples (Furnham, Tan, and McManus 1997; Singh 1993; Singh and Young 1995; Streeter and McBurney 2003); not coincidentally, 0.7 is the average WHR of *Playboy* centerfolds (Singh 1993).

The studies of WHR tend to draw heavily on evolutionary ideas about human preferences because, evolutionary psychology argues, BMI or body volume (Tovée et al. 1999, 2002) and WHR (Singh 1993, 1994; Singh and Young 1995) are reasonable markers of mate quality and therefore the most consistent and likely universally regarded indices of female body attractiveness. A main proposition of this approach is that men's responses to bodies and other physical markers have evolved to help them make better reproductive choices, and that markers such as BMI or WHR index something critical about a person's genotype or phenotype (Buss 1989). The basic assumption is that men use their responses to bodies as a basic heuristic to answer the question, Is she fertile? (Low 2001).

For example, overall body fat has been suggested as a cue of fertility because ovulation, pregnancy, and lactation all draw on it (Ellison 2003; Frisch 1990); a lower WHR is thought to index fertility, youth, and health because it is associated with lower age, higher estrogen, and lower parasite loads respectively (Singh 1993). If the basic propositions of this evolutionary argument hold—that male and female mate preferences have evolved to select for reproductive success, and that fat or body shape is one critical index of that potential—we should expect to see universally similar positive responses to some types of bodies (for example, a preference for a low WHR or an aversion to skinny or obese bodies).

But studies from diverse societies have challenged the universality of a male preference for relatively small-waisted women. In China, men have been reported to prefer a more curvaceous WHR of 0.6 (Dixson et al. 2007), and Ugandan men to favor a ratio of 0.5 (Furnham, Badmin, and Sneade 2002). In other countries, men prefer a much higher WHR (0.8 or 0.9), including Matsigenka horticulturalists of Peru (Yu and Shepard 1998), Shiwiar horticulturalists of Ecuador (Sugiyama 2004), Hadza hunter-gatherers of Tanzania (Marlowe and Wetsman 2001), and Cameroonians (Dixson et al. 2007). Marlowe and Wetsman (2001) argue that Hadza men select a higher WHR because they prefer fatter women, and this makes good sense given that food shortages are common in their environment. A follow-up study (Marlowe, Spicella, and Reed 2005) found that Hadza men specifically preferred women with lower WHR when viewed from the side (that is, they preferred buttocks that protruded).

These authors have argued against a measurable universal WHR preference among men, positing that men tend to prefer the WHR typical of younger women in their own society (ibid.). Others have found that body mass more than WHR shaped men's responses (e.g., Cornelissen, Tovée, and Bateson 2009). This finding might suggest that men's preferences for women's bodies go beyond WHR. Several studies support this notion. When Swami and colleagues (2007) showed men in Britain, Portugal, and Spain pictures of women's bodies with known BMI and WHR, what the men judged attractive—although they preferred slimmer figures—was more closely related to BMI than to WHR. The same finding was reported for a comparative study of Greek and British men (Swami et al. 2006).

Such evolutionary literature presents an intriguing possibility: that in selecting a mate, perhaps men in a given ecological setting prefer the body type that is the more difficult to attain, particularly one that requires more effort, skill, and resources (such as money). Men in societies experiencing food shortages or other nutritional stress would therefore tend to prefer higher BMI or plumper women, while those in toxic food environments (where excess calories are easy to acquire and slimness requires work) would have slimmer ideals

(Scott et al. 2007). In general terms, studies of less Westernized groups with less stable food supplies support this notion.

Some researchers have interpreted this idea in light of an "environmental security hypothesis" (Pettijohn and Tesser 1999) that suggests that the idea makes adaptive sense because it helps us make good mating choices (Nelson, Pettijohn, and Galak 2007). In this model, "it is not culture that shapes the individual, but instead, as the environment alters the individual, it is the individual who shapes the culture" (ibid., 202). This is a very different way of looking at the relationship between body ideals and culture than we see in most of the more traditionally focused ethnographic studies we turn to next.

6

Big-Body Symbolism, Meanings, and Norms

To explain how and why body image preferences might vary cross-culturally and why slim ideals may penetrate more readily or forcefully in some groups and places than in others, we need to understand and acknowledge cultural variation in the symbolism of big bodies. We can assess the critical issue of how this symbolism relates to the cultural and social context more broadly only on a case-by-case basis with some ethnographic depth. One reason for the variance in people's attitudes toward large bodies is that the value placed on bodies culturally, that is, the symbolism imbued in the bodies, differs by culture.

One of the classic examples of cultural differences in how people understand the symbolic meanings of fat bodies comes from a South African public health campaign in the 1950s (Gampel 1962, discussed in Brown and Sweeney 2009). White public health workers put up two posters as part of an anti-obesity campaign. One depicted a large woman beside a heavily loaded truck with a flat tire. The caption read: "Both carry too much weight." In the other, a thin woman swept dirt under a table while a much larger woman leaned against it. "Who do you want to look like?" the caption asked. Zulu observers, equating largeness with wealth, knew the answer to the question was the bigger woman. It was clear to them that the larger woman had servants to do her sweeping and, as the first poster showed, so many possessions that her truck was unable to hold them all.

Mary Douglas (1970) was one of the first anthropologists to develop the idea of the body as a symbol. In this way of thinking, the body is a text written with a culture's social meanings, and to fully decode those meanings one needs to be an expert reader of or in that culture (Reischer and Koo 2004). Drawing from Douglas, many scholars understand the body as a means of symbolic representation, expressing core social and cultural values (e.g., Ritenbaugh 1982). For example, Balsamo (1996, 78) calls the body "a site of inscription, a billboard for dominant cultural meanings." In the West, the dominant social messages about fat bodies are overwhelmingly negative and applied forcefully to the individual. In many other societies in which anthropologists have specifically investigated this point, no negative values exist for big bodies for women, and in some, positive values attach to big bodies for women—as feminine, sexy, fertile, powerful, valuable, and morally good.

In Belize, for example, where bodies are seen as immutable and God-given, body shape and size are accepted as natural and not interpreted to mean anything in particular about an individual, according to Eileen Anderson-Fye. Her 2004 study of body image and eating disorders in young women in Belize provides an example of a social setting in which body size is not particularly socially salient as a key aspect of beauty, even though women are exposed to the full range of Western ideals. San Andrés, the only town on a large cay in the Caribbean Sea, sees the most tourists of any part of Belize and is highly dependent economically on tourist dollars. U.S. television is widespread and contact between locals and visitors in San Andrés is greater than in most other tourist destinations in the region. Anderson-Fye was especially interested in how susceptibility to eating disorders might be tied to exposure to Western body ideals. She interviewed eighty young women using three different interview protocols—open-ended narratives (where the informant helps shape the direction of the interview), survey-style interviews (where the questions are the same for all respondents), and clinical interviews (commonly used by health practitioners in diagnoses). She also ran focus groups (a good way to elicit information about norms), applied a standardized psychometric test for disordered eating (the EAT-26), and had the young women complete a standard body image scale (the scale she used is not specified). Finally, she spent considerable time in informal settings with many of the girls, such as at parties and events.

What Anderson-Fye found using these methods is that these young women felt that body shape, rather than body size, was central to their attractiveness. In particular, girls valued a Coca-Cola body, the traditional hourglass shape that is curvy at the top, slim waisted, and bigger and curvier at the bottom. They laughed about not wanting a "diet Coke" shape, straight up and down like the sides of a can. They understood body size, by contrast, as relatively unchangeable, a natural outcome of family heritage or a gift from God. Thus, for San Andrés women, trying to change their body's size was unimportant and a waste of energy. It was not possible to be too thin or too fat; shapely beauty was about how you adorned what you had, rather than how you shaped it to fit some ideal. Many of the young women enjoyed participating in local beauty pageants, whose winners came in all sizes and ethnicities, reflecting the community's pluralistic ideas about beauty. Also not surprisingly, these girls were highly accurate in identifying their body size on the body image scales. Anderson-Fye summarizes:

Beyond the ethical imperative toward self-care, controlling and changing the body simply was not possible in significant and lasting ways. . . . For the San Andranas, control was exerted through adornment, dressing to emphasize the Coca-Cola shape, hairstyling, and makeup application. While the emphasis on beauty for women remained strong, the means to achieve it involved working with what one had to highlight qualities considered beautiful rather than disciplining the body into a uniform ideal. Beauty, then, consisted of multiple ideals sharing certain uncontrollable and malleable characteristics, on both an everyday level and the pageant stage. (2004, 570)

Another example of a society that does not take a negative view of fat bodies is Jamaica. The ideal body in the communities Elisa Sobo studied in the late 1980s is well rounded and plump, and plumpness is not only aesthetically pleasing but also valued for its associations with positive attributes such as fertility, youth, sexuality, high status, happiness, power, and health. Many Jamaicans see big bodies, like full breasts and erect penises, as charged with life and vitality; they are delicious and "sweet." Thinness has negative cultural connotations for Jamaicans, marking infertility and meanness in a society where having children and enjoying social support and cooperation are core social values. In this context, weight loss indexes stress or illness, because happy and healthy people are fat (Sobo 1993).

In these Jamaican communities, families who share wealth and feed each other are considered good—no one will be rich and no one will be thin when things are as they should be. Thus, being too rich or too thin is an index of things gone awry, a sign that someone is being antisocial, mean, or stingy (Sobo 1994). To be plump is to show through your largeness that you are part of a caring family and have good, reciprocal social relations. To be called big is a mark of respect. To be called skinny implies that one lacks power and social commitment, and represents social and physical decay. Thinness symbolizes a lack of nurturance, an absence of connection, vibrancy, and procreative power. Because eating builds the big bodies Jamaicans value, parents feed children, couples feed each other, and kin feed the group; the growth of one's body thus symbolizes love from one's family and lover. To grow thin is to let the world know that the love is gone or the relationships with one's family have broken down. Smith and Cogswell (1994) suggest that this Jamaican ideal of plumpness remains revered partly because of its contrast to foreign preoccupations with thinness. That is, the idealization of plump becomes a point of resistance to external forces.

Pacific Island cultures are similar to Jamaican culture in that the body is traditionally viewed as a symbol of the community rather than of the individual. The body is culturally understood as an expression of how the community is faring, and hence as a collective achievement or failure. Becker's work in the central Pacific nation of Fiji is a particularly clear exploration of this idea: how the community inscribes its values onto big bodies, and how and why the individual goes along with this. Her interpretation of the ethnographic data is that the body is less an expression of self than a "community resource for expression." That is, the symbolic messages of the body convey something essential about the social group, not about the individual. Thus, Fijians gain social prestige by the bodies they associate with, not just by their own body (Becker 1995).

In Fiji, the body does not express personal identity or achievement; it is a way for people to integrate themselves into the community in a society where belonging to a community is critical. Fijians are attentive to weight loss because it can represent a failure of the community to take care of its members, and this reflects badly on everyone. Thus Fijians, like Jamaicans, understand bodies in terms of their embeddedness (or lack thereof) in collective care. They see large bodies, as long as they are not the result of hoarding, as well-tended bodies that signal a proper, ongoing, generous flow of goods and services and that are linked to social rather than individual material gains (Gremillion 2005, 17). This view helps explain in cultural terms why Fijians might be unlikely to see overweight or moderate obesity as a problem, to want to moderate their weight, or to understand why anyone would not want to be fat.

Starting in the late 1980s, Anne Becker conducted an extensive ethnographic study of the connections among bodies, sense of self, and social values in a Fijian village near the mouth of the Sigatoka River, a rich agricultural area on the main island of Viti Levu. A decade later, she returned to Fiji to follow up on her study and especially to test how exposure to television, introduced to Fiji in the intervening period, might be shaping conceptions of bodies. In the first study, Becker (1995) did traditional participant-observation in the village and also administered a series of surveys on diet and body shape attitudes to 301 adults. She documented that women selected body ideals in the middle of the range, similar to those selected by both Kenyan and British women in another study using the same scale (Furnham and Alibhai 1983). Also like the Kenyan women, the Fijian women were more accepting than British women of larger bodies at the top of the scale. Becker also demonstrated through qualitative analyses that Fijian women's bodies and sense of self, in contrast to those of women in the West, are rooted in the collective and the sense of community rather than in the individual.

In Becker's later study, she used narrative data transcribed from semi-structured interviews and focus groups with Fijian high school girls and found that body aesthetics had changed substantially in the preceding ten years, and that the identities of women had been reshaped in some fundamental ways. In particular, an identity shaped by Western television images and role models in which self-presentation was key was starting to replace (or at least hybridizing with) the construction of personal identity through nurturing others. To many of the high school girls, social advancement was now tied to looking a particular way. As one participant said: "I want to become like those women [on TV, in magazines]. They are very slim and tall, that I'm losing my weight, that I am trying to be like them" (Becker 2004, 541).

In much of the classic ethnographic work by anthropologists looking at bodies, such as Becker's study in Fiji, we see a strong emphasis on understanding how bodies are used as symbols to express core cultural values. In all societies, body morphology is deployed as a way to express and reinforce core social values, and thus the interpretations of body size convey qualities of the individual well beyond the aesthetic. In this way, the body is part of the cultural order of society, a site at which cultural tensions or conflicts can be displayed. The acceptable and ideal body is prescribed culturally, and so our bodies are shaped by culture as we struggle to meet those ideals.

Social constructionist approaches draw on this idea of the body as social symbol or social metaphor, but also consider the production of meanings in society and how we manage ourselves and each other as social beings, such as how people construct preferences through interacting with each other. This approach begins with a central assumption: whether being obese is a problem is much less important than how it becomes regarded as one (Honeycutt 1999). Our bodies can act to reflect and maintain the social order, and in this way, the body can have agency, meaning that not only does it express social meanings, but also it is active in creating our social worlds and social meanings. Understanding the body as socially active, awarding it agency in shaping how we act and how we understand the world, is often referred to as "embodiment" (Csordas 1990). Thus, bodies not only project powerful symbolic messages but also participate in the creation of social values and meanings, and at every level these can be contested. A central construct in this approach is that humans make choices and affect each other, even when structural influences constrain their choices. It emphasizes that human actions are determined by human creativity and interaction, not just by structural circumstances (Maurer and Sobal 1999, 3–4).

A number of researchers have applied this approach in examining the ways in which our bodies are tied to each other and to broader social processes in a dynamic way. In this sense, obesity's definition as a problem reflects the way collective norms are shaped and expressed. The idea of embodied human experience—that we experience the world from the confines of our own body—has influenced medical anthropology during the last few decades and is a useful approach for thinking about how cultural messages shape, and are shaped by, our bodies and the values we place on them. We can also use the idea of embodiment to think about the body as a sociocultural (rather than a biological) construction.

Much of the medical anthropology research in this vein has addressed or focused on women and gender issues (Singer and Baer 2007, 94). Emily Martin, in her classic text *The Woman in the Body* (1989), explains how Western medical traditions tend to understand the body as a passive machine managed through medical intervention. This explanation fits well with ideas common in the West about obese patients as difficult and noncompliant in how they relate to their doctors and the medical system.

Industrialized nations also offer examples of social settings in which big bodies are symbolically viewed as good and beautiful. Emily Massara's ethnographic study conducted starting in the late 1970s included in-depth interviews and intense participation in the lives of nine technically obese Puerto Rican women in Philadelphia. The study was focused on understanding cultural factors related to the rapid weight gain common at that time among Puerto Ricans in one neighborhood in the north of the city. Puerto Rican migration to the area had mainly occurred in the post–World War II era, predominantly for jobs as farm workers. Massara found that the community interpreted mild or moderate levels of obesity as reflections of tranquility and satisfaction in life, health, good appetite, and well-being, whereas thinness was reviled and feared. The women expected to gain weight—a good twenty pounds or so—after they married. Failure to gain weight was interpreted as a clear sign that a woman's husband was not doing a good job providing for her, and thus called his breadwinner status and manhood into question. Similarly, weight gain in pregnancy was attached to the idea that eating what one craves and desires keeps the baby healthy. Massara concluded that many women were very happy to be—or aspired to be—overweight, given its positive cultural connotations. In this context, being skinny or having noticeable weight loss was invariably understood as indicating misfortune and loss, such as malnutrition or chronic and potentially life-threatening disease. In looking at the slim figures on the female body image scales, women said, "She is dying," or "She is thin like an invalid." As one of her participants said:

> When I was heavy I had an easy life and nothing happened to me. When I lost weight, people said: "You're so skinny! What happened to you?" So many people told me fat I didn't look bad and I looked better that way because I had shape. Now I am down and out. People don't understand your problem. . . . I saw a friend yesterday I hadn't seen in a long time. She said, "How did you lose so much?" (Massara 1989, 141–142)

Rebecca Popenoe's study of the Azawagh Arabs (eastern Moors) in Niger, West Africa, is one of the most detailed ethnographic examples of a society in which extreme levels of female fatness are highly valued. Popenoe, like Sobo and Massara, applied the standard ethnographic method of participant observation. She spent many days with women in their tents, watching and chatting.

In this Islamic, semi-nomadic society, fatness is so desirable that girls begin their fattening rituals at about age five. Fat bodies are considered attractive and sexy. A full, plump body is understood as soft, pliable, seated, immobile, and feminine, a contrast to the valorized male body, which is hard, erect, and mobile, a reflection of the careful distinction between male and female roles and forms expressed in Islam. Women work to develop not just big bodies but large buttocks, fleshy thighs, fat folds around their stomachs, and stretch marks on their arms and legs. Female relatives force-feed Azawagh girls large bowls of millet porridge and milk—food thought to be best at fattening—for several years before puberty to build the full, abundant, luscious body that men and women both admire, a practice thought to hasten puberty and hence womanliness, sexuality, and marriageability. Popenoe makes a convincing case that perceptions of luscious big bodies persist among the Azawagh even as they come into increasing contact with Western ideas, because they are tightly tied to core cultural values and social structures implicit to Azawagh Arab society. The critical symbolic meanings attached to big bodies are an integral part of social life and thus are perpetuated.

> The appeal of fatness is also grounded in a fading nomadic world in which milk is still the most valued of foodstuffs, flowing rich and white from animal udders and invested, so to speak, into the lush, moist fat of women's bodies. In this way the milk that comes from the animals men own and manage is transformed into the stuff of women's status and desirability, and ultimately into the breastmilk that nourishes future generations. Milk and women's bodies encapsulate value, both material and symbolic, for the community as a whole . . . ; women mediate a translation of material culture into social value through their bodies in a way that enhances that value immeasurably. (Popenoe 2004, 8, 189)

The Azawagh case is also a good example of how people in some societies come to associate the beautiful with the good, just as fat and unattractive have become entwined conceptually in the West.

> The Arabs of the Azawagh region considered it impossible to imagine that where I came from women did not want to be fat; indeed, I think they never believed my protests to the contrary. . . . When I asked people directly about the aesthetic, they almost invariably answered "because it is beautiful." To both men and women it seemed a rather nonsensical thing to come asking questions about. The aesthetic, like beauty aesthetics everywhere, seemed so obvious and natural to its adherents that they had little incentive, indeed little cause, to reflect upon it. (Popenoe 2004, 7)

Popenoe's Niger study is also a particularly good example of how the concept of agency can be applied to analyze the ways that women's fatness—and its connections to ideas about desire, kinship, health, religion, and sexuality—can be explained within wider social structures and in line with cultural logic. The process of fattening in Niger is a way girls can work toward the fulfillment of their religious duties, as those responsible for producing the next generation of faithful members. This process in many ways mirrors the almost religious discipline of Western women who work to slim their bodies. As Popenoe (2004, 192) explains: "Female fatness among Azawagh Arabs is thus not only expressive and symbolic of fundamental cultural tenets, but also provides women with a powerful way of exercising agency over their own lives." By becoming and being big and immobile, the Azawagh woman gains social solidity and proves she is able to control her own desires and deny her own interests in favor of those of her community and society.

Historically and cross-culturally, a range of societies like the Azawagh practice cultural fattening (rituals designed expressly to make people fat, because fat bodies have greater social value). A number of groups in Nigeria, Tanzania, Uganda, and Kenya use fattening huts to prepare women for marriage, making them as attractive as possible by plumping them up (Malcolm 1925; Roscoe 1923). In the fattening rooms of Nigeria's Annang (Brink 1989), the bride's plump body symbolizes the affluence and status of the girl's family that will extend to her husband's family after the marriage occurs. Before marriage, women are placed in confinement so they can avoid any undo exercise and eat high-quality foods, such as expensive meat. Generally, fattening is a practice only the wealthy can maintain, and the poorer members of the society cannot participate in the rituals. In sub-Saharan Africa, a part of the world that still suffers from widespread undernutrition, preference for large bodies appears to have some historical depth. It is maintained today in some particular cultural contexts, where its value remains so socially profound that it tends to resist the global trends spreading with mass media and the market economy.

Fat, Ugly, and Bad

By sharp contrast with societies that value the social messages conveyed by fat, fear and loathing of body fat and conversely the veneration of slimness are powerful, pervasive ideas in the industrialized West. These are most fanatically expressed in Northern Hemisphere, Protestant cultures (de Garine and Pollock 1995). The label of obesity is laden in English with almost exclusively negative social meanings and with a loss of mind-over-body control (de Garine and Pollock 1995; Turner 1984). Study after study shows obesity and fat to be perceived as unattractive, unsexy, unhealthy, and—for women—unfeminine, and associated in people's minds with a host of character or personal failings: weakness of will and lack of control, stupidity or low IQ, lack of hygiene, and self-indulgence. The large and fat are thus characterized as "lazy, sloppy, dirty and worse . . . destroying grace and delicacy" (de Vries 2007, 61; see also Cordell and Ronai 1999; Dejong 1993; Grogan and Richards 2002; Stunkard and Sobal 1995). Obesity is thus not simply a physical state; it also has been ascribed moral meanings. In mainstream U.S. society especially, a tightly woven cultural relationship exists between fat as unattractive and unhealthy and fat as morally degenerate and socially inadequate. In contrast, thinness is associated with beauty, intelligence, wealth, attractiveness, class, grace, health, discipline, and goodness (Caputi 1983; Moreno and Thelen 1993).

Mimi Nichter's (2000) ethnographic research with teen girls in Tucson, Arizona, provides a very readable example of how these ideas about fat and thin become a critical part of how girls talk, woven into the very heart of how they understand and relate to themselves and each other. Nichter and her team spent three years talking with 211 early teenage (eighth and ninth grade, approximately thirteen to fifteen years of age) girls at two middle schools and two high schools in Tucson. The study used a combination of standard interview techniques (surveys where everyone answers the same set of questions and open-ended formats), records of what girls ate, and annual measurements of their height and weight. The team also conducted a series of focus groups with girls, talking with small groups of friends from the same social set (prep, mod, skater, or stoner), because mixing social circles inhibited open discussion. The surveys and one-on-one interviews provided the information on individual eating behaviors and attitudes, while the focus groups were important for getting at generalized attitudes toward weight and eating. They supplemented the formal parts of the study with participant observation at the schools, hanging out in the cafeteria and around school to observe what girls were talking about and eating.

The group found that these teen girls had profound concerns about their weight as it shaped their sense of self and their relationships with others. The "perfect girl"—blond, five feet eight, 100 pounds, long hair, white teeth, perfectly dressed—was a widely held ideal that resulted in the girls devaluing themselves, as almost no one could live up to it. In this socially competitive, fat-concerned world of teenage girls, the overweight White girls were acutely aware of the stereotypes applied to them—as jealous of the skinny girls, lazy, lacking self-respect, and less attractive to boys (or even running the boys off). The negative moral and competitive connotations of fat were clearly voiced, for example: "I mean, when we don't like a girl, we won't be like, 'She's a bad person,' or 'She's mean,' or 'She's a liar,' we'll say, 'Oh, she's ugly,' or 'She's fat,' or 'Did you see her thighs?'" A slim and popular girl said: "Who wants to be seen with a fat person? I mean I try to avoid really large people. . . . I just try and stay away from them" (Nichter 2000, 36). In contrast, African American girls in the study refused to diet, and they drew purposefully on alternative, nondominant messages about bodies from family and community that were more accommodating of nonnormal sizes.

A common speech ritual for the White girls was to open with, "I'm so fat" (even when not), to which the ritual reply was, "Oh, no you're not!" This "fat talk," as Nichter calls it, is not idle chatter but serves a variety of important social purposes: as an idiom of distress to express a sense of stress or being out of control, as a call for support from friends, and to affirm group membership, to mitigate discomfort, to maintain a social competitive advantage over others, to reinforce the importance of fitting in and looking like everyone else, to call attention to one's flaws before others do in the socially competitive world of middle and high school, and to connect and build rapport through a shared concern of avoiding fat. However, girls also talked to themselves in this way, speaking to their mirrors in a sort of inner dialogue, assessing how well they met or (usually) failed to meet the body ideal.

Nichter summarizes the results as follows: "Discussing their bodies opens a floodgate of emotions in young girls, including jealousy, envy, rage, and alienation. Such feelings are silenced by some, whispered by others, and shouted by a few. By age fourteen and probably much, much earlier, many white middle-class girls have surmised that social competence comes from conformity, with striving toward the elusive ideal of perfection. . . . The image of the ideal is always close by, lurking like an inescapable shadow in the background of girl's lives" (Nichter 2000, 44).

The negative connotations of fat as unhealthy, unattractive, and immoral are not the only set of social messages attached to fat in thin-preferring societies, as we shall see, but definitely the dominant one. In many ways, the slim idealism so evident in the West can be understood more fundamentally as a "fear of fat" that has some historical depth in Western thinking (Littlewood 1995). In the West, fatness and fat symbolize immorality and challenge core cultural values. Cross-cultural studies suggest that the strongest anti-fat biases are found in countries like Australia, England, and the United States, where the two cultural ideas of individualism and thin idealism intersect. Individualism is the idea that people are individually responsible for what happens to them in life, and thin idealism a concept that places high value on thin bodies (Crandall et al. 2001). These cultural ideas apparently contrast with those in countries such as India, Turkey, and Venezuela, where collectivism is valued above individualism and where fat bias or stigma tends to be much less obvious or profound, even if people also tend to have relatively thin body ideals (ibid.).

Antifat messages seem to target and have their greatest impact on women. For many women, there are clear messages that nothing is worse than being obese, and death might be a reasonable price to pay to achieve thinness. The results of an online survey by Schwartz and colleagues (2006) suggest that for many U.S. adults, early death or divorce, loss of a limb, or even blindness would be preferable to being obese. Furthermore, the slimmer the respondent, the more drastic the apparent trade-offs he or she was willing to make to avoid obesity (see table 6.1). Curious about this somewhat stunning statistic, in the last year I have been working with several student collaborators with data samples of university students and more general samples of adults in Phoenix, using a variety of techniques. These have included both in-person and online interviews, and included a matched-pairs method where participants selected the conditions they would rather endure or be known to have versus obesity and versus all other conditions (for example, "Would you rather be obese or be known as a racist?"). The results were similar in overall impression to those of Schwartz and colleagues, in that regardless of the approach we used, participants tended to rate obesity as less preferred against a host of both stigmatizing and disabling conditions. For example, some half of 1,400 respondents in one round of data collection said they would rather die five years sooner than be obese.

Going from obese to not obese can precipitate a massive change in people's sense of self, especially for women. In one study, 100 percent of preoperative, morbidly obese people considered themselves unattractive and 77 percent said they were depressed. Fourteen months postoperatively, 100 percent said they felt attractive. Before surgery, 40 percent of participants said they always or often experienced all sixteen types of prejudice or discrimination listed on the survey. (Items included statements like "I do not like to be seen in public because of my weight," "I feel that children and adults stare at me critically in restaurants and shopping malls," and "I feel I have been treated disrespectfully by the medical profession because of my weight.") Postoperatively, between 87 and 100 percent of participants answered "never" to the same items (Rand and McGregor 1990).

These ideas about fat as failure link to a broader Western core value that attributes any form of failure (dropout, divorce, poverty) to a lack of motivation to succeed and thus a failing of the individual (Simmons and Rosenberg 1971). Maddox, Back, and Liederman (1965, 32) explain that "in a society which has historically been suffused with a Protestant Ethic, one characteristic of which is a strong emphasis on impulse control, fatness suggests a kind of immorality which invites retribution. Correspondingly, the reduction of overweight and the avoidance of the contagion of gluttony implies self denial, which ought to bring appropriate rewards, including good health." In most of the West, a person with a slim (and increasingly trim and toned) body is understood as having greater self-sufficiency, autonomy, control, and strength of character. Obesity is the inversion of these core values, a loss of control and thus a highly negative reflection on the self in a society where the self is central. This idea that obesity symbolizes a loss of self-control is widely apparent in the public health literature, which suggests that obesity in contemporary Western society is a product of individual lifestyle decisions, within one's own control and easily reversible with the application of sufficient self-control, discipline, and willpower.

TABLE 6.1

**Reported Desire of U.S. Adults to Avoid Obesity,
by Trade-off and BMI Category**

	Body Mass Index (BMI) Category of Respondent				
	Under-weight	Normal weight	Over-weight	Obese	Extremely Obese
To avoid obesity, I would be willing to:			*(% answering yes)*		
Give up 1 year of my life	71.9/	57.4/	41.6/	30.5/	34.3/
(Mean no. of years people would give up)	8.93	4.81	2.75	2.23	2.45
Be divorced	65.4	35.7	27.4	20.1	23.9
Be unable to have children	47.1	27.0	23.6	22.8	22.8
Be severely depressed	52.3	20.8	8.1	9.3	10.7
Be alcoholic	42.9	19.8	12.5	5.6	6.1
Lose a limb	22.4	7.0	3.9	2.2	3.0
Be blind	16.3	5.0	3.2	2.1	3.6

Source: Drawn from the results of an online survey of
4,283 adults (Schwartz et al. 2006, table 3).

A number of studies have shown that more news articles commonly convey the idea of obesity as a personal responsibility than offer structural explanations for obesity, although references to personal solutions for obesity dramatically outnumber references to personal responsibility for its causes (Kim and Willis 2007; Lawrence 2004).

This notion of personal responsibility emerges clearly even in science. For example, Edwards and Roberts (2009) suggest that people's failing to maintain their BMI at the carbon-appropriate level is a partial cause of climate change. They calculated the difference in greenhouse gas emissions from two theoretical populations with standardized heights and the same daily activities. Members of one population were normal weight, similar to the United Kingdom in 1970; members of the other had a 40 percent rate of obesity (mean BMI of 29), comparable to the United Kingdom in 2010. The authors estimated that the overweight population required 19 percent additional megajoules per day of food energy per person on average to maintain their basal metabolism and provide energy for basic daily activities (12.3 versus 10.3 MJ). That 19 percent difference represents an additional 0.27 gigatons (GT) per year in global greenhouse gases (mainly carbon dioxide) from the extra food production needed. They also estimated that overweight people would create higher transportation-related emissions because they are heavier to transport and use up more energy if walking because the effort is greater. The authors totaled the greenhouse gases related to car travel, air travel, and energy needed to walk and came up with a figure of greenhouse gas emissions related to obesity of between 0.4 and 1.0 GT of carbon dioxide equivalents annually. Estimates of total human emissions of CO_2 vary greatly based on how they are calculated but fall in the range of 25–50 GT annually (Intergovernmental Panel on Climate Change 2007). In the late 1970s, when obesity was still relatively uncommon, a study suggested that if everyone in the United States reached their optimal weights by dieting, the reduction in food consumption would save the equivalent of 1.3 billion gallons of gasoline (Hannon and Lohman 1978). The implications of these studies are clear: overweight people do damage to us all.

Given that these ideas about personal responsibility for being overweight are implicit in our scientific understandings as well as our cultural ideas, it is perhaps not surprising that large people perceive discrimination and that there is evidence of systematic bias against them in many areas of modern life. Experimental studies show that people are less likely to apply negative value judgments to obese persons if they are told that the individuals are obese for a medical reason beyond their own control, such as a thyroid condition (Crandall 1994; Crandall and Martinez 1996). The core idea of personal responsibility for obesity diverts our attention from structural factors (like poor food environments) that put people at risk in the first place (Farmer 1999). It also gives people more personal agency than they have under certain conditions (for example, poverty) and shapes the way in which individuals are blamed and authorities fail to do anything about the structural shapers of that suffering (sometimes termed "social suffering").

Two Western ideas in considerable tension with each other that influence how we think about obesity as morally bad are that our bodies are "to be escaped" and "to be worked on" (Becker 1995, 33). To Becker and others such as Emily Martin who study the body as a social metaphor, the body is fundamentally alienated from sense of self in the West, meaning it is highly objectified and seen as something one should be able to control (Becker 1995; Martin 1989). Obesity in the West is thus highly stigmatizing not only because it symbolizes a loss of control, but also because the overweight body is seen as a direct reflection of the self within it. Self-restraint is one core value in Western society that affects our aversion to fat bodies (MacKenzie 1985). Thus, among many Western women, the idea of "being good" and "doing the work of being slim" are entwined. For example, it is not uncommon to hear a woman say, "I was good today," in reference to watching what she had eaten that day or her going to the gym.

In the West, bodies have become one of the most dominant, preferred symbols of the "self" (Becker 1995, 33). A big body symbolically represents an "unrestrained" or "uncontrolled" self, one who is morally weak and lacking self-discipline. Other characteristics applied to the self within a fat body include ineptitude, laziness, indulgence, and insufficient "working on" the body. By the same token, a slim, toned, correctly sculptured body symbolizes that the right work has occurred, and it communicates adequacy, discipline, control, and beauty to others. Becker (1995, 36) summarizes:

> The modes of body cultivation have proliferated through the various industries designed to transform the body's appearance. . . . Breast augmentation and reduction, liposuction and collagen injections. The intensity and extremity of this investment in resculpting the body are testimony that "no price is too great, no process too repulsive, no operation too painful, for the woman who will be beautiful." . . . In short, vanity has been transformed into a virtue in which "creation of self" is the "highest form of creativity"; . . . this stems from the commodification and objectification of the body within consumerist late-capitalist society.

Perhaps one of the best examples of body cultivation, now increasingly widely performed and accepted, is bariatric surgery designed to remove or bypass most of the stomach so that massive weight loss results. Failing to distinguish between the body and the self, the Western approach now views the size and shape of the body as the symbol of the moral status of the individual (Bordo 1993; Reischer and Koo 2004).

The effect of this symbolism on women is often profound, as studies by Jenny Carryer (1997, 2001) show. In a sequence of interviews with nine significantly overweight New Zealand women over a period of two years, Carryer found overwhelming suffering tied to their internalization of all the negative social and cultural meanings of fatness. Clare, one of her participants, said: "We feel quite different to other people. We feel overweight; we always think they're looking at you being overweight. You have these guilt feelings if you eat something you shouldn't. You sort of feel uncomfortable, your body just feels bulky. . . . And if you happen to put on some weight you feel depressed and if you take it off it makes you feel good." Another participant, Heather, said: "And then you do a double take when you see yourself in a shop window and you think my God I am as big as that and you feel yeah, a little bit disgusted—really disgusted" (1997, 87, 114).

These women expressed disgust for their own and others' large bodies, as well as their belief in the moral messages of fat. For example, one participant said, "If you are fat you are lazy" (Carryer 1997, 117). As a large woman herself, Carryer felt she could connect both emotionally and intellectually with her participants, and engaged in an ongoing dialogue with them that included discussing the conclusions of her work. In summary, she found: "Being a fat woman is to experience a prolonged, personal battle with the body; . . . the battle is enacted in a social context which is the site of remarkable consensus about the personal culpability of fat people for their bodily largeness; for women in particular the sanctions are especially powerful." And Carryer notes: "I can only argue that for participants in the project 'fat acceptance' seems a remote dream" (1997, 108).

Susan Bordo, a widely cited postmodern feminist scholar, has written about how women's bodies in the Western tradition are seen to encase and thus express the self. The development of anorexia nervosa and bulimia, she suggests in her 1993 book *Unbearable Weight*, are almost inevitable physical reactions to cultural ideas about a slim body as representing mastery over one's desires. She shows in a series of essays how this idea is expressed in—but also shaped by—cultural images, such as advertising. Bordo understands the female body as migrated from nature to culture through time, to the point where it can be altered by such practices as surgery and dieting and has emerged as a constant site of conflict. Dieting is thus a patriarchal practice of discipline in which the body is both subjected and the subject, trained into the feminized, docile form. Bordo uses media examples to show how the message conveyed is that "we can 'choose' our own bodies" using surgery, diet, and exercise to sculpt our ideal image of self—a hollow promise, because for many the ideal is unattainable. Thus the message that everyone can attain perfect slimness if they would only make the effort allows us to judge negatively those who do not, and therefo· promotes shame and guilt (Gard and Wright 2005, 160). In other words, a core requirement of Western culture is that women must take responsibility for disciplining their bodies to meet the cultural norms of femininity.

> In this context women with large bodies are stigmatized in ways that profoundly affect their personal and public lives. In the first instance they are blamed for exceeding the boundaries of their bodies, they are said to have "let themselves go," which suggests they have no self-control. Fatness is seen as the result of self-indulgence, as a rejection of the structures of a society that expects self-denial and the repression of desire. In addition, from a medical perspective, the fat woman is blamed for "causing her own fat" as she is unable to manage her own body and therefore able to be subjected to the control of others, such as doctors and health professionals; . . . it is social expectations around femininity that shape the stigmatization of women and the ways they internalize these. . . . This is not a requirement of men, large bodies can be powerful bodies, and appropriately masculine. (Gand and Wright 2005, 161)

Thus, "in 'capitulating to desire' fat women are seen as . . . breaking the rules, and culture's immediate reaction is to punish them" (Hartley 2001, 66). That is, society at large feels that "if the rest of us are struggling to be acceptable and 'normal' we cannot allow them to get away with it; they must be put in their place, be humiliated and defeated" (Bordo 1993, 203).

Millman's 1980 book *Such a Pretty Face* suggests that U.S. women with large bodies tend to distance themselves from their bodies, to feel they are disconnected—or want to be—from their unwanted bodies. Jenny Carryer in her study of overweight New Zealand women finds that the idea of "embodied largeness" accurately describes how Western women understand and act in their big bodies. "Suffering" is the word Carryer chooses to express the all-encompassing and constant concern over their embodied largeness that seems to penetrate every aspect of overweight women's lives—work, marriage, family, and leisure. Carryer, like many other feminist scholars interested in women's bodies, is strongly influenced by Foucault's theory of discourse (see Foucault 1972 in particular), which emphasizes the centrality of discourse, the set of ideas revealed by how we speak, what we do, the texts we write and read, and the institutions we create and to which we are subject. In his view, discourse shapes and reflects how we live and how we experience. The idea of power is central to this theory (medicine provides a good example of a dominant, almost unlimitedly powerful discourse about obesity, including the "fat is dangerous" message), as is the idea that "truth" and "meaning" are constantly contested. (It should be noted, however, that a set of competing or converse cultural ideas exist in the West related to big bodies, including one that equates big bodies with rebellion and the rejection of social norms and self-acceptance.)

A fascinating aspect of Western symbolism about fat bodies is that overweight women appear to internalize it and hence accept the core messages at least as much as, and maybe even more than, others. A number of studies have found that obese people tend to agree with the majority cultural norms about the meanings of their size (Joanisse and Synnott 1999). Honeycutt's (1999) interviews with eighty-nine large women who were active dieters, pro-fat activists (such as members of the National Association to Advance Fat Acceptance, NAAFA), or neither revealed that most women in all three groups failed to challenge conventional definitions of body obesity, and in many cases they reified or promoted them. In other words, the women had internalized the cultural norms that negatively judged them. One key aspect of the sociocultural construction of fat aversion in the West is that women, fat and thin, appear to be complicit and active in perpetuating and even promoting the thin ideal and fat stigma:

Women themselves become the ultimate "body police" by internalizing the cultural imperatives of the thin ideal. Women are encouraged to modify and monitor themselves and other women in a never-ending process of body-surveillance to conform to the culturally acceptable body image, even at the expense of their health. . . . As "bearers of their own surveillance" through the internalization of sociocultural discourses, women are conceptualized as colluding; . . . [however] not all bodies are so "docile" and . . . resistance to the thin ideal through female agency can create the "social spaces" where alternative discourses form and challenge the dominant discourse; . . . the possibility exists for women to break free from the "social" bars that constrain and construct them. (Germov and Williams 1999, 125–127)

The possibilities for fat women to "break free" include accepting their size, becoming political activists, joining support groups, and framing themselves in relation to feminine ideals that use criteria other than body size. The Health at Every Size Movement takes specific issue with current views of fat bodies and the approaches of obesity treatment (Gaesser 2003) and promotes nurturing self-acceptance and being at peace with one's eating; the movement defines health as what emerges from a meaningful, satisfying, and comfortably active life (Robison 2006). In particular, proponents challenge what they describe as a traditional weight-loss paradigm that equates thin with health and happiness and overweight with lack of self-discipline (ibid.).

Of course, the media are implicated in all this pervasive negative messaging. Not just advertising but also television programming is pro-thin and fairly anti-fat. To examine how messages about being fat or thin are delivered in various types of media, studies have applied content analysis, a formal method that tests the content of media or other texts to determine, among other things, what core messages they are communicating. One such study, which looked at 1,211 cartoon programs and some 4,000 cartoon characters since 1930, found that over time not only has the number of overweight characters declined but also overweight characters are more likely to be portrayed as unhappy, unintelligent, unattractive, or aggressive and as eating junk food, and less likely to be the "hero" (Klein and Shiffman 2005). Another study found that in popular childhood videos and books, thin female characters were much more likely than overweight female characters to display positively valued traits such as being kind, happy, sociable, and successful. Overweight characters were more likely to be cruel, evil, or unattractive, were never involved in romantic attachments to thin characters, and were often shown seeking food or eating (Herbozo et al. 2004).

An analysis of nineteen unanimated sitcoms broadcast on children's channels in the United States, such as *Sabrina the Teenage Witch* and *Hannah Montana*, turned up different results (Robinson, Callister, and Jankowski 2008). Taking four episodes of each show recorded in one calendar month, two people independently coded the gender and ethnicity of each character listed on the program website as a main character with a recurring role, and then used body image scales to rate each as very thin, thin, average, overweight, or obese. They also coded the main characters based on factors such as portrayed intelligence, leadership, appearance, and popularity. The researchers found very little difference in how overweight, obese, normal, and underweight characters were portrayed, except that overweight characters were slightly more socially marginalized.

The Social Consequences of Obesity:
Stigma, Prejudice, and Bias

The concept of stigma—negative social attributions applied to individuals because they are labeled with a specific disease or illness—is also useful for thinking about overweight and obesity because of the contextual and cultural variance in what is socially devalued and valued in regard to body size and fatness. Until now, I have been using the term "stigma" in a generic sense to refer to negative social value placed on excess overweight. The notion of stigma is also used in a more particular way in medical anthropology to refer to the process by which the reaction of others interferes with individuals' normal identity and causes them to be socially discredited (Goffman 1963). According to Erving Goffman's schema, obesity is a potentially socially damaging condition when stigmatized because its presence is so obvious and so difficult to mask. He discusses how an individual becomes devalued or shunned because of a disability or illness that makes them abnormal or different. Stigmatized conditions often trump all other social features of a person, creating intense suffering (Becker 1998).

Obesity as a chronic condition is obvious and thus highly public, core to people's social identities. In Western society, being very overweight can be termed a "master status"—a shaper of identities that overrides everything else about a person; one is identified as deviant before any other identities are recognized (Becker 1963, 33). A core message here is that characteristics perceived to be controllable are the responsibility of the person bearing the stigma, which can in turn influence how an individual reacts to and copes with the negative attitudes of others. Often part of coping with a stigmatized condition is finding ways to socially manage it so that others do not respond so negatively to it. Wearing full-coverage clothes or telling people that one is dieting are two coping mechanisms that, at least in the West, seem to make a difference to how negatively others react to obesity (Zdrodowski 1996; see also Maurer and Sobal 1999).

Weight stigma is so tied to identity that it produces a global devaluation of the individual attached to the trait. By the same token, many Western women who lose large amounts of weight undergo a profound and dramatic process of identity change in which they often reassess who they are and how they relate to others, taking on a new status and set of roles (Rubin, Schmilovitz, and Weiss 1993). Similarly, as women gain weight they can undergo a fairly complex process of reframing their central identity to become a "fat" person (Degher and Hughes 1999). But the characteristic in question (being fat) is of itself neither innately creditable nor discreditable—what stigmatizes one set of people may emphasize the normalcy of the other. What counts is the degree to which a community considers the characteristic deviant.

Certainly, the stigma associated with overweight and especially obesity in contemporary Western societies is potent and profound, and the social costs to the obese individual are correspondingly high. Puhl and Heuer (2009) recently summarized all the published studies on prejudice and discrimination related to obesity, as an index of manifestation of that stigma, and the evidence of prejudice and bias is overwhelming. Obese adults are less likely than thin adults to get accepted at the best universities, are paid less for the same job, have greater relative difficulty getting hired, are perceived to do a worse job once hired (independent of performance), and are less likely to be promoted and more likely to be terminated. Obese people report being more likely than thin ones to be on the receiving end of derogatory humor and pejorative comments from family, colleagues, and strangers alike. Overweight children are also less well liked than their average-sized peers, more likely to be bullied and to bully others, and more likely to suffer from depression (Janssen et al. 2004; Sjoberg, Nilsson, and Leppert 2005).

Good evidence of systematic and widespread bias against the overweight and obese also exists in health care settings. One study of some 620 U.S. physicians found that more than half of them labeled obese patients as awkward, ugly, and noncompliant, and a third characterized obese patients as weak, sloppy, and lazy. Moreover, most of the physicians attributed the patients' obesity to aspects of their own behavior, such as an unhealthy diet (Foster et al. 2003). Similar findings have been reported for physicians and other health care professionals in France, the United Kingdom, Australia, and Israel, with many respondents attributing characteristics to the obese such as laziness and lack of willpower (Bocquier, Verger, and Basdevant 2005; Campbell et al. 2000; Fogelman, Vinker, and Lachter 2002; Harvey and Hill 2001). Similar bias turns up in studies of fitness professionals and dieticians, who have been reported to label fat people as lazy, unattractive, eating too much junk food, and able to lose weight if they would just put in the effort (Chambliss, Finley, and Blair 2004).

These attitudes may well contribute to less support for weight loss in obese patients. A range of studies has shown that physicians often believe obese patients are beyond treatment or have low expectations for patient success

(Puhl and Heuer 2009). And it may not be any surprise then that overweight and obese patients perceive themselves subject to prejudice, inappropriate comments, unsatisfactory treatment, and ambivalence by health care professionals (Puhl and Brownell 2001).

A number of studies have documented weight bias in close relationships, including romantic relationships, especially for obese women. One recent study asked 238 U.S. university students to rate a personal advertisement from a woman seeking someone to date (Smith et al. 2007). When the woman was described as "fat" or "overweight," the ad elicited more negative responses from students than did more positive or objective descriptors ("full figured" or "197 lbs"). Recent research has shown that one's closest family members may exhibit prejudice against us if we are obese. In a study that examined the experience of weight stigmatization in a sample of more than 2,400 overweight and obese adult women, the women most frequently cited family members as the source of negative messages (Puhl and Brownell 2006). In another study, parents were shown pictures of children (one not overweight, one obese, and one disabled) and instructed to tell a story about each picture to their child. The least positive stories (with failure-ridden endings and the lowest achievers) related to the overweight picture. Other studies have shown that weight teasing by parents is common for adolescent boys and girls, and that parents provide more financial aid to their leaner offspring, even controlling for parental education, income, ethnicity, and number of other children (Adams, Hicken, and Salehi 1988; Crandall 1995; Eisenberg, Neumark-Sztainer, and Story 2003).

Studies looking at the effects of obesity and stigma related to it on close relationships and social support have produced more mixed findings. A study of 3,656 U.S. adults found little difference in the quality of relationships with spouses, colleagues, or friends reported across weight categories (Carr and Friedman 2005). Studies from Finland and Germany have shown no clear differences in loneliness or subjective well-being between the obese and not obese (Dierk et al. 2006; Sarlio-Lähteenkorva 2001). Wherever stigmas do exist, however, they seem to impact women more than men (Puhl and Heuer 2009).

What is perhaps more fascinating about the process of stigmatization in relation to obesity is that those who are big in a fat-stigmatizing society tend to accept and internalize the cultural norms about obesity that preclude them from being fully socially valued, condemned to "eternal stigmatization in their own eyes as well as those of society" (Albon 1981, 8; but cf. Siegel, Lune, and Meyer 1998). Based on a grounded analysis of the transcripts of interviews with twenty-nine women who were members of a national weight-reduction organization, Degher and Hughes (1999) found that women used a variety of means to "socially manage" their stigmatized obese identities once these were internalized. The most common method was to avoid social situations in which fat became socially problematic and hence stressful, such as looking in mirrors or going to public swimming pools. Others ignored it, or tried to, as one woman shared:

> You know, most of the time I am pretty happy. I don't even think about being fat. It only happens when something happens, like having to fly, and not being able to fit in the seats and having to ask for a seatbelt extension, that I start to think about it again. If I had to think about it all the time, I think I would kill myself. (20)

Others responded to negative social cues by sporadically eating more, perhaps in many cases as a self-punishing response. Still others worked hard to overachieve in other aspects of their lives, for example, by being the best possible friend, mother, community volunteer, or employee. Some, especially those who had been obese since childhood, saw excellence as the only way to gain social acceptance. Yet another strategy was to engage in what the authors call "compliance" behavior, where the women went along with dieting efforts to placate others, were willing or eager to be the butt of the joke or to be the "jolly fat person" (commonly portrayed on television), or willing to degrade and humiliate themselves.

The final coping strategy Degher and Hughes highlight is what they call "accounts," which are stories the person told to explain their large size in ways that shifted the responsibility away from self. These included "fat stories" about weight-inducing conditions such as hormone problems, medication, illness, poor socialization, marriage, and parenthood; and also "eating stories" about how personal tragedies or other stressors led them to gain weight. Even when this strategy was used, though, there is some evidence that the individuals socially managed the negative labeling through active resistance. In a study of the life history narratives of ten overweight women, conducted in a somewhat similar fashion to that of Carryer's study of New Zealand women, Cordell and Ronai (1999) discuss how women resist some aspects of the negative social messages by constructing their identities in ways that defy the messages and the deviant status afforded to the obese. Women may describe themselves as attractive, sexy, and in control of their bodies, and try to index to others that they don't hate their bodies while avoiding behaviors attached to the "jolly fat person" stereotype.

This discussion helps explain some of the possible social bases of the higher rates of depression and other mood disorders such as anxiety that are associated with obesity. Furthermore, it may explain why these disorders are much higher among women, the better educated, and majority ethnic groups in the United States, where obesity rates are lower and thin preferences and fat abhorrence are more evident (Simon et al. 2006). This makes good theoretical sense, but few empirical studies have explored the connections between obesity and culture in such terms.

The medicalization of obesity, discussed in chapter 2, is a double-edged sword with regard to obesity stigma and the way in which people react to obesity in the West. On the one hand, the very application of the term "obesity" has shifted some emphasis away from the failings of the individual and removed some (although not all) of the moral undertones associated with terms used earlier, such as "plump," "fat," or "corpulent." Among medical practitioners, the individual-responsibility model seems to be that most often expressed. Pool suggests (2000, 36) that most believe the etiology of obesity to be partially bio-logical and physiological, in that everyone eats too much sometimes but some—for genetic or developmental reasons—have a harder time maintaining or losing weight than others. Among those who do research on obesity and those who design and implement prevention or interventions related to obesity, a notable tension exists between the idea of personal responsibility and obesity preven-tion focused on public policy, built environments, and social change (Lawrence 2004).

On the other hand, medicalization draws attention in a concerted, even frantic way to the "dangers" of obesity. The model most common among lay people that holds the individual responsible for losing control over weight gain also means that overweight adults and children are expected to meet fairly specific prescriptions in order to be healthy and "get better" from their medicalized condition. In this model, if parents fail to help their children lose weight, they are denying them a normal life by denying treatment and possibly even committing child abuse. In the United States, a number of court cases have determined obese children to be neglected by their parents; in a Texas case, decided in 2002, parental rights were terminated for a four-year-old boy who weighed more than 136 pounds. The decision would probably have gone differently if there was widespread ascription to the structural basis of obesity (such as poor food environments or poverty more generally).

Cognitive, Comparative Approaches
to Culture, Stigma, and Obesity

Exploring symbolism and agency, such as through analysis of people's narra-tives, can help us figure out how social structures and the underlying power relationships (Who controls whom? Who benefits?) might act upon and be resis-ted by the obese individual. Similarly, analysis of how the symbolism of large bodies varies helps us think about why people have quite different reactions to larger bodies, although our understanding of the broad patterns of cultural vari-ation remains extremely limited. By contrast, a cognitive view of culture under-stands it as based on sets of logical rules and organized domains of knowledge that can be systematically elicited; this view applies a scientific approach to its analysis. Current cognitive approaches, such as those I apply in my research, tend to focus on how cultural knowledge is distributed within domains, such as what is shared among different people (the "culture") and what implications this creates. One of the reasons I apply this approach is that it provides a solid basis for comparing cultural variation across groups, and it is arguably the method of culture most compatible with broader-scale modeling. Given the trend toward dynamic modeling as a way to increase the interpretability of data, which is taking off in the social sciences, this approach is likely to gain increasing traction in the years ahead.

Some of the key comparative questions we can ask using systematic forms of ethnographic research include: Is the powerful stigma attached to obesity in the West globalizing, as bodies grow bigger everywhere so that more and more people are affected by it? If there is some globalization of the negative cultural messages about obesity, which ones tend to dominate globally? Are some societies that are undergoing large increases in obesity rates thinking in quite different (even positive) ways about the increasing numbers of large bodies? Are there still societies that do not stigmatize fat in any way? Do people understand the causative bases of obesity differently or similarly around the world (acknowledging that many of our views in the West about obesity are culture bound, not science based)?

In the previous chapter, we discussed how slim ideals are now seemingly globalized, at least as reflected in the finding that women in most parts of the world on average want to be smaller than they currently are. Colleagues and I set out in the summer of 2009 to determine if fat stigma appeared to be spread globally as well. We used a fairly simple tool, a cultural statements survey, to collect comparative data about how people were thinking about obesity in a range of diverse settings, from large, highly industrialized and globalized cities to isolated, rural locations. We currently have samples from eleven places, including three places (American Samoa, Eastern Africa [Tanzania], and Puerto Rico) historically glossed as "fat positive" in the ethnographic record (see appendix D for sample sizes and characteristics). The samples represent a wide range of ecologies and economic development, different levels of obesity risk, and different levels of education. In each place we administered the same survey of sixty-eight statements about bodies and obesity (translated into the local language), to which each respondent gave only a true or false response. Appendix D contains a discussion of how we selected the survey items, which cover perceptions of the causes, consequences, and characteristics of obesity.

A consensus analysis of the data from these eleven samples (see appendix D for an explanation of this method) revealed a shared cultural model across all the countries, and emphasizes a number of core ideas about bodies that we have generally associated with the West: that obesity is an individual responsibility, that people are fat because of what they do or don't do rather than for structural reasons, and that fat is bad and slim is good. A shared cultural model is the set of beliefs about the world that together represent an underlying understanding about it. This does not mean that everyone agrees with every belief in the shared model, or even that everyone agrees with most elements of the shared model. Rather, the shared model is the underlying set of ideas that more people agree about than disagree. Not everyone necessarily has the same pattern of beliefs, and one can be "outside" in terms of one's perception of something like obesity, or one can be "inside" and have a set of ideas about obesity that overlaps considerably with the shared model.

We see the same types of themes in each of the individual country samples (see appendix D for the answer key for each group), and comparing the findings across the sites suggests several important conclusions. First, ideas about the social and health value of thinness appear to be almost universal. Second, ideas about the negative value of fat predominate but are not universal. Third, education is a powerful determinant of the spread of anti-fat ideas. (However, because the demographic measures in our study are somewhat crude, it is also possible that education is acting as a proxy for something else, such as people's socioeconomic status or the extent of their engagement with global media.) Finally, the most interesting conclusion is that the cultural group that individuals belong to or where they live are not the most significant predictors of how they think about body size and obesity.

When we look at how normative body mass index plays into these cultural norms by looking specifically at the relationship of people's competency scores to their BMI, we find that people with high BMIs have very normative ideas (close to the shared model) about big bodies (figure 6.1). In other words, they are likely to have negative ideas about obesity, and to view obesity as a personal responsibility rather than as the result of structural factors. That is, there is no clear relationship between BMI and cultural competency scores, within and across groups. This means that having more overweight and obese people in a population does not necessarily influence directly the group's normative response toward big bodies, and that anti-fat ideas do not necessarily diminish as more people gain weight within a group. These findings agree with the general findings of the qualitative studies discussed earlier, such as Honeycutt's (1999), which suggest that many overweight and obese people tend to be as accepting, or even more accepting, of the negative meanings applied to their fat. From our study, we see evidence of this finding across a variety of cultural and ecological settings, not just in Western or Anglo samples.

One of the most important findings of this comparative study is that it shows evidence of some globalization of fat stigma. Twenty-three of the sixty-eight statements in the survey tool applied socially discrediting ("People are overweight because they are lazy") attributions to large or fat bodies. When we convert the responses across the study samples into a "stigma score," the results

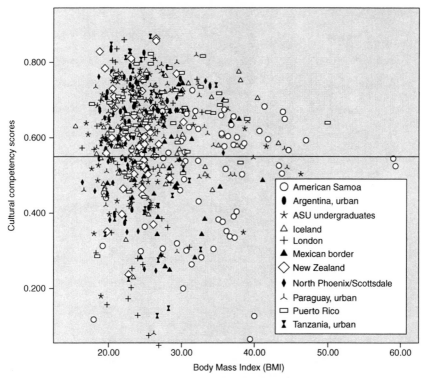

FIGURE 6.1 Relationship of respondents' cultural competency scores to their BMI in samples from eleven countries. Cultural competency was measured by an individual's knowledge of culturally correct answers about obesity. The line at 0.55 indicates basic competency; 0.100 is the highest level.

are stunning. Fat stigma is readily apparent in all samples, and at a relatively consistent level and range (see figure 6.2).

Interestingly, the stigma scores are higher in middle-income developing countries, including those that the ethnographic record would suggest tend more toward the fat positive, such as Paraguay, American Samoa, and Mexico. As noted, overall the cultural models tend to suggest norms whereby one is overweight due to one's own failings, fat is very unhealthy, and some negative social attributions associated with fat are understood. However, overt discrediting on the basis of overweight is not normatively considered acceptable in some countries, while it is at least more openly stated in others.

This systematic approach to measuring how cultural variation is related to obesity gives us new, replicable, context-meaningful ways to start thinking about the variation in the way people think about obesity (and related phenomenon such as food or exercise), and to model that variation. Given the interest generated among colleagues and graduate students by the projects we

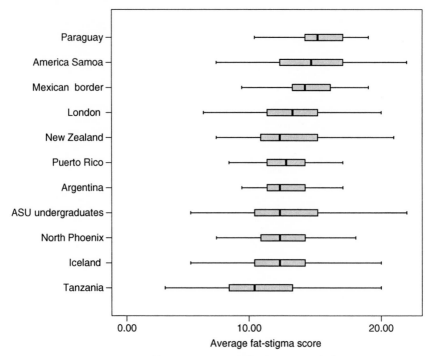

FIGURE 6.2 A comparison of fat-stigma scores of cultures sampled in 2009. For each culture, the shaded area represents the occurrence of scores between the 25th and 75th percentiles, with the average score falling in the middle. The dark vertical line in the shaded area represents the median score; the extended horizontal line indicates the range of scores.

have been conducting, I suspect that in the next few years we will see a proliferation of this type of research focused on obesity and related domains, as well as efforts to use such techniques as agent-based modeling to better generalize results and explain when and why things tend to be so locally specific. This research will greatly enhance not only our ability to theorize culture and obesity links but also to design and test obesity interventions in new, better, and more generalizable ways.

We are also using agent-based modeling to integrate this information about stigma with data about obesity within neighborhoods, such as food environments. If we can then also combine all this with high-quality, detailed, local ethnographic approaches, such as seen in the work of Rebecca Popenoe on the Moors or Anne Becker in Fiji, then our understanding of the cultural bases of obesity, and ultimately of obesity more generally, will be advanced substantively. And with this, we will improve our capacity to leverage understanding of the cultural bases of obesity in ways that have the best chance of helping people live healthier lives.

7

Conclusion

The Big Picture

The emergence of a fat-rich body as a norm represents a profound biological shift for our species. The conditions that allow the accumulation of excess fat in a systematic way within a population—sustained amounts of readily available, calorie-dense food and sedentary lifestyles—were absent for the great part of human history yet now define most of the industrialized world. As low- and middle-income countries continue to urbanize and increasingly depend on global food systems, obesity rates will continue to rise.

Looking forward, how worried should we be about the global rise in obesity? Is our concern slightly hysterical, or entirely well founded? Colleagues in the offices down the hall from me at Arizona State are variously attempting to solve problems of pandemic influenza, antibiotic resistant forms of tuberculosis, and safe, potable drinking water. In this context, it is hard to sell obesity as a crisis issue. Several scholars have made the argument that the discussion of obesity is greatly overblown and ridiculously panicked (Campos 2004; Gibbs 2005). They note that the health effects of obesity are not as grave as the government and public health science claim, so that what should probably be framed as a personal issue has been demonized as a sociopolitical one through stigmatization of fat (Kersh and Morone 2002; also see Johnston and Harkavy 2009). The greed of the weight-loss industry that benefits from our cycles of weight loss and gain is also indicted as fueling the fire (Campos et al. 2006).

When we weigh the epidemiological evidence (see chapter 2), it is not clear that being overweight or obese is of itself inherently unhealthy, and in some cases (especially for the elderly), it may even be the most healthy state. Lifestyle factors (especially level of sedentariness, quality of diet, and stress levels) are much more important than weight in shaping overall health. A recent observation that we hear little about is that Americans are becoming shorter on average and losing height relative to those in Europe (Komlos and Baur 2004). Why aren't we concerned about our decreasing height relative to weight, which of course makes us fatter too?

Yet the increasingly observed developmental links between epigenetic factors (such as gene-environment interactions in utero) and how we metabolize food and store fat (discussed in chapter 3) mean that the rapid increase in levels of child obesity globally could be particularly worrisome. Childhood obesity tends to predict an elevated risk of obesity in adulthood, and childhood obesity rates are much higher now than they were when today's overweight adults were themselves children. Furthermore, since obese adults compared to not obese adults tend to raise children at greater risk of obesity, there may be an additional generational effect that has not fully emerged yet.

More critically perhaps, the convergence of undernutrition with overnutrition that is occurring in a number of countries will magnify the likelihood of being overweight as well as its negative health effects. This phenomenon is likely to spread over the next decade or so, as poorer nations become increasingly integrated into global economies and as urbanization and industrialization accelerate. Moreover, these poorer nations have limited health care resources to begin with, and thus virtually no capacity to deal with the chronic disabilities often associated with obesity. If this is the case, we have an economic, as much as a moral, imperative to invest heavily in reversing the current trends. Otherwise, the potentially massive health and economic costs of obesity threaten to engulf entire national economies and reduce quality of life in the years ahead (Popkin 2009). Viewed from this perspective, obesity is clearly a big deal. Many government and nongovernmental agencies and foundations (including Centers for Disease Control and the World Health Organization) agree. They classify obesity as one of the major global public health challenges today and are investing increasingly large amounts of money into alleviating it.

If we decide the obesity epidemic deserves attention from a public health perspective, then what are our best options for addressing it? The examples of the failed Five-a-Day and Fit for Life campaigns discussed in the opening of the book (where massive investments to get people to eat less and exercise more came to nothing) show that most traditional public health campaigns that attempt to get the population to lose weight have had, at best, equivocal results. A recent review of family-based interventions found the results just as uncertain, although the design of the studies had enough weaknesses that it was impossible to determine exactly what impact the strategies had (Berry et al. 2004). A review of child-focused studies reached much the same conclusion (Campbell et al. 2001).

Why the failures? Based on the research discussed throughout this book, we can suggest several different answers. First, we have to recognize that being obese is in many ways a problem only because we collectively agree it is. As we saw in the data on thin ideals and fat stigma from a variety of countries presented in chapters 5 and 6, obesity is understood at a basic cultural level as a symbol of failure to maintain self and health. Our ideas about fat being bad are so fundamental to our social and cultural values, and so profound and pervasive, that they are barely ever questioned (Ronai 1997). Obesity has become increasingly defined and discussed within the confines of disease in the West, and this is shaping how we respond to it. We thus believe that our primary care physicians, not our legislators and city planners, should be charged with identifying and addressing any obesity problem, and we increasingly turn to individual medical fixes (such as surgery) to deal with obesity rather than demanding the reorganization of our cities to encourage collective exercise. In this way, we are saying the body must be changed because it offends our culture, not our culture that must be changed to accommodate the body (Joanisse and Synnott 1999). In the larger picture, it would probably be productive to take a leaf from the fat-acceptance mantra and disassemble the idea of being big from the idea of being unhealthy and diseased.

Alternatively, if we take the perspective of human adaptation presented in chapter 3, our biology has been honed over millions of years to efficiently deposit adipose tissue when excess calories and fat are available, and to hold onto it. This makes sense when food supplies are erratic, which characterizes the environments we lived in for most of human history. It means, as a species, we are primed to get and stay fat if at all possible, both in terms of how we react to food psychologically and metabolically and what happens when we exercise. In this view, the basic reason we are gaining weight as a species is because we now live in ecologies and have lifestyles that are highly obesogenic (fat promoting), compared to those we have lived in through the vast majority of human history (Eaton et al. 1988). Thus, weight loss or maintenance is at the most basic level a fight against our own evolved psychological and physical selves. From this perspective, we would expect food and built environment interventions to be a productive way to proceed. However, as discussed in chapter 4, to date there is no clear empirical evidence that changes in food environments actually reduce overall obesity rates in a community. In the absence of clear evidence that demonstrates the exact pathways between genetic underpinnings and obesity on the one hand and environmental factors on the other, we are stuck focusing primarily on the role of behavior in how we design evidence-based interventions. Explicating those pathways should therefore be our main focus moving forward.

In addition, so many aspects of our culture, not just our physical ecologies, are obesogenic, and the pathways by which these become manifest as weight gain also need to be much better understood (Johnston and Harkavy 2009). There are myriad culturally constructed barriers to a svelte population tied to our core values in the West; the drive for and desirability of consumption and the value placed on individual choice and responsibility are just two. The desire for easy thinness underwrites a massive diet and exercise industry (which benefits from its own lack of success), and our basic values shape how we choose to shop, get to and from work, and what we do with our leisure time. So, being slim is "to swim against the current of cultural forces that lead to fatness; it is a culturally constructed obesogenic environment" (Brown and Krick 2001). Viewed this way, obesity is a much harder public health challenge than addressing swine flu or other major infectious diseases such as malaria or tuberculosis. It requires fundamental social, ecological, and technological changes that go against the grain of what makes us human at this particular point in time. As with the Pima example, discussed earlier, massive institutional transformation across all the requisite domains within communities and neighborhoods is probably the only thing that will make a profound difference to expanding obesity rates in most of the world.

Where successful obesity intervention has occurred, it tends to be in small pockets where culturally specific tactics have been developed and applied (e.g., Wilson 2009). One way to improve this strategy is to recognize that most community-based approaches to obesity that purport to be culturally aware often highly conflate ethnicity with culture, an approach that will miss a lot of the most important tailoring that should be done. The consensus statement by the American Diabetic Association (Caprio et al. 2008) cited earlier, for example, recites the differences in exercise and eating habits based on ethnicity with almost no recognition that there can be as much variation in how people view the world within these socially constructed categories as there is between the categories. Our data show considerable variation within and across groups in how people conceptualize weight, as well as in how they think about food, eating, and exercise (see chapter 6). Two people from the same town and of the same self-reported ethnicity with the same body weight can have quite different beliefs about weight and food, and these views may also change over time. The conflation of ethnicity as culture in much of the public health approach to obesity mistakenly assumes that people within the same group tend to think alike and statically.

Another way to improve obesity interventions is to shape them with an eye to the *dynamics* of culture (Emmons 2000). Cultural knowledge does not occur in a vacuum; it is highly shaped by a wide array of factors, including whom we tend to talk to, how we identify ourselves, the social and economic opportunities open to us, and the built environments in which we live. We need to develop conceptual models that can incorporate those inherent and complex dynamics.

In summary, obesity interventions generally do not work because most address obesity in a narrow, reductionist way. Obesity is a complex, multifaceted, deep-rooted part of the contemporary human condition that resists simple, singular, quick, or easy fixes. Because it has stemmed from fundamental social, economic, and ecological changes our species has faced over the last few decades, only sustained and fundamental examination of those conditions is likely to do much about it. If powerful and broad global processes shape obesity, global solutions may ultimately be needed (Sobal 2001). Unfortunately, there does not seem to be the political will to create global solutions to obesity—at least not compared to, say, climate change.

Perhaps partly for this reason, Johnston and Harkavy (2009, 2) argue convincingly that the pragmatic approach to obesity that deserves highest priority is one that thinks globally but acts locally, an approach that "conceptualizes obesity as a highly complex, ill-structured, real-world problem that requires ongoing, collaborative research and action involving the collaboration of individuals from a variety of academic disciplines and community members in a working partnership to solve this urgent problem." No single fix will resolve the problem, and no one approach will be sufficient; in fact, the problem itself is constantly changing.

The question of how we address obesity right now poses some challenges. First, interventions in the proximate factors that shape obesity—nutrition, exercise, and body image—occur in relative isolation from each other. This is hardly a recipe for success, since they are tied together, as well as to obesity risk, in complex ways. Second, community buy-in to prevention and intervention efforts is critical to their short- and long-term success. Third, because obesity results from chronic, not acute, conditions (whether at the proximate or ultimate levels), one-step or one-shot solutions are unlikely to be effective. Instead, potentially the most effective way to deal with obesity is through long-term commitment to address the problem from multiple perspectives at the neighborhood level. Any such long-term efforts will need widespread buy-in and a shared sense of purpose and commitment across stakeholder groups—local government, local health care, local community, and academic partners—to address obesity from multiple intersecting perspectives.

A good example of this approach is the set of initiatives undertaken by the University of Pennsylvania and the local West Philadelphia stakeholders, community members, and institutions, especially local schools (Johnston and Harkavy 2009). West Philadelphia is comprised of predominantly Black neighborhoods, with double the national rate of families living below the poverty line, and higher than the national average rate of childhood obesity, both overall and for African Americans. Over the last fifteen years, these initiatives have included efforts to develop urban agriculture and to expand service-learning opportunities through the university to improve food knowledge and food environments in the community. Other efforts have focused on increasing options for physical activity, as well as work with area schools to improve specific nutritional knowledge and general problem solving in the curriculum.

These initiatives have successfully increased fruit and vegetable consumption among schoolchildren in the area (Johnston and Harkavy 2009), but no measurable data yet show that obesity risk in this community is going down. However, the framework that has been set up, which emphasizes collaborative, real-world problem solving as a partnered enterprise across key players (local neighborhoods, schools, city planners, and researchers), combined with an ongoing, long-term commitment to address the problem within a specific community, seems the approach most likely to succeed over the long haul.

This approach also importantly recognizes that obesity needs to be better acknowledged as a social justice issue in policy and in practice. An analysis of who is fat in the contemporary world, we have seen, often shows that disadvantages tend to get heaped on those at the bottom of the social ladder. In the United States and other industrialized nations, obesity risk is decidedly high among minorities and especially in low-income areas (compounded by the fact that many minorities are concentrated in low-income areas). A fair society should pay much more attention to how amenities (such as parks, walkable neighborhoods, and healthy food sources) are distributed in our communities, a shift that should make a difference to those most at risk.

These considerations strongly influence how we manage our current projects in South Phoenix, a low-income, mainly Mexican American community near downtown. I have spent several years working with a group of other social and applied scientists to develop a participatory framework for the project in which we identified obesity as an issue that community members were especially concerned about and ready to talk about. We have developed a network of researchers, community agencies, and community stakeholders (such as clinics, the Parks Department, and food banks) to tackle the problem in an ongoing and roughly coordinated way across all levels—individual, family, school, neighborhood, and institutional. This initiative is a little different from others I have been involved in because it is framed with an evolving agenda, designed to adjust to whatever new challenges and problems arise. The intersecting activities our collective is working on include understanding the extent and nutritional impacts of food environments, including urban agriculture; collecting baseline data to characterize the metabolic profiles of this specific target population; looking at how the economic downturn is impacting food availability; examining park access and how that is affecting exercise; and doing ethnographic evaluations of the child obesity interventions being conducted by various agencies within the community. The underlying principle of the project is that obesity is a complex, multifaceted, and evolving problem, and our approaches to dealing with it will need to keep that principle front and center if they have any hope of working effectively with our community partners to make any difference over the long term.

One interesting wrinkle is that we have flipped the standard questions about why people are overweight, and instead asked how some people maintain a normal weight in obesogenic environments. In other words, if environments such as low-income, inner-city neighborhoods are often fundamentally obeso-genic, with poor access to fresh, healthy food, low walkability, and few options for safe and pleasant exercise, then how do some individuals manage to avoid overweight and obesity? This puts a much more positive spin on community-based studies—if we can focus on what people are doing that works to keep them from becoming overweight and then extend that to people who are over-weight, the solutions will more likely be feasible, reasonable, and meaningful in the specific context. For example, social sports such as amateur soccer leagues are popular for men in this community, so encouraging more men to play soccer may help combat weight problems.

So far, we have talked mainly about obesity and what to do about it from a health standpoint. Most interventions ignore the stigma attached to obesity, and the damage it wreaks on obese individuals' sense of self, psychological well-being, and opportunities. Obesity is arguably the only remaining socially and legally acceptable form of discrimination in the United States. The cross-cultural

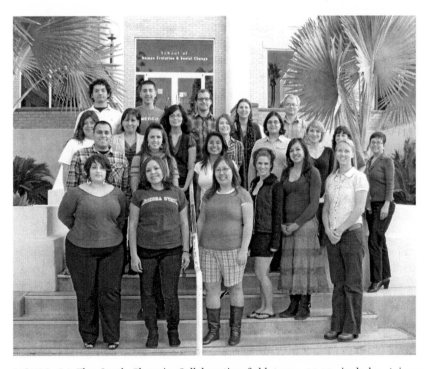

FIGURE 7.1 The South Phoenix Collaborative field team, 2009, includes Arizona State University students from South Phoenix who lead the data collection effort, social and applied scientists, and community stakeholders who guide data collection and dissemination.

Photo courtesy of the School of Human Evolution and Social Change, Arizona State University.

record clearly shows nothing innate to the human condition to make us feel revulsion toward fat, and in many places big, beautiful, and fabulous have gone together.

To me, one of the most interesting questions in the area of culture and obesity is whether and how this fat stigma is spreading globally. On the surface, it is counter-intuitive that people would tend to be fat in the places where fat is most devalued. I suggest that three key reasons may explain this seeming paradox. First, as noted, it is difficult in contemporary environments to be slim, requiring resources (time, money, and knowledge) not available to everyone—one of the reasons slimness has social value. Second, even if people identify a slim ideal or recognize fat stigma, not everybody cares about or finds the slim ideal or fat stigma salient to them—such attitudes vary culturally but also by age, stage, gender, and ethnicity. Finally, in an obesogenic environment, even those who want to be slim and have the resources to be slim may not make slimness their highest priority. Investing in a career, spending time with family and friends, or looking after one's children, for instance, might trump this desire.

What might be the implications of a global rise in fat stigma, given how socially damaging they can be? Body image studies report a global shift toward increasingly slim body ideals. In every place comparable metric data has been collected, women report they want to be slimmer than they are. Although comparable studies of a few cultural pockets, such as the Azawagh Arabs (chapter 6), might produce a different result, but it is safe to say that the value placed on slim bodies is well on the way to being global. What is less clear at present, mainly because it has not received much attention, is whether the socially crippling stigma attached to obesity is spreading as well. In our study of Samoan women in the 1990s, we found them taking on thin ideals without the fat stigma, and the results of much more recent data across a variety of countries also suggest that fat stigma is not an automatic corollary of either the spread of thin ideals or the increase in levels of obesity at the local level.

Still, we see that people with cultural models that incorporate stigmatizing ideas about fat (that fat is an individual responsibility and that it is bad and has moral meanings) are present in societies (such as Samoa) where fat was acceptable or attractive traditionally. This is worrisome, because the damage obesity does to quality of life in industrialized nations is often as much or more in the social than in the health domain. Looking forward, we have to worry not only about the health and economic costs of an obesity explosion in the developing worlds, but also about its other impacts on quality of life if the stigmatizing effects of fat also expand into a much wider range of cultural settings. Given that much of the suffering associated with obesity is social in origin, it is horrifying to think of the large number of people in developing countries, right now perfectly happy with their bodies, who might soon learn the self-disgust and experience the social rejection that comes with Western anti-fat ideas.

The cross-cultural record can also provide an important perspective, because our negative response to fat is highly enculturated, which means that it is entirely possible to unlearn it. One can look at the massive change in social attitudes to same-sex sexual orientation or to working women over the last century to see how extreme change in such fundamental ideas is possible. A focus on the cross-cultural record (rather than on only the ethnographic particularities of any specific case) critically shows the inherent flexibility in how people perceive bodies. We are starting to understand which aspects of fat aversion or avoidance may be universal and how these might be globalizing or being resisted, and to think more clearly and comparatively about the anti-fat values omnipresent in the West. Our studies have in this way highlighted how bizarre Western anti-fat bias is, viewed comparatively and historically. We now need research that highlights and explains the variability between cultures.

What other future areas might interest those researching obesity in the context of culture? One interesting development for culture-obesity studies is the move into more explicit and methodologically sophisticated studies of the dynamic relationships between culture and obesity, probably best done using agent-based modeling. This shift will allow us to better address the inherent causal complexity in the construction of obesity, which is not accessible in traditional forms of data analysis (such as standard statistics). We are also expanding our studies to look at how obesity knowledge (such as fat stigma) is distributed in people's social networks and how that shapes the way they view and respond to their bodies.

One other related question that we are working on concerns the pathways between obesity, culture, and depression. There is evidence that being overweight leads to depression (and especially that weight loss reduces depression), and that depression also contributes to weight gain and obesity. However, there are also likely to be some complex relationships between social networks and how obesity and depression are associated. For example, it is hypothetically possible that overweight people who are around thin people and who have thin-preferring cultural models are much more prone to obesity, especially if their cultural model matches that of others around them. This hypothesis is based on the assumption that the proximate social conditions related to fat stigma should shape psychological as well as physical status and also mediate the dynamic connections between the two. Importantly, from the perspective of biocultural anthropology, depression rates are understood as a responsive marker of levels of social stress experienced by individuals (Hadley and Patil 2006; Hadley, Brewis, and Pike 2010; Pike and Borovoy 2004; Pike and Patil 2006), and higher levels of depression are used to index high levels of social stress within a given group. When we consider the social costs of obesity (such as stigma and prejudice) and acknowledge that women appear to be most subject to these, it seems important to take account of depression as we conceptualize the possible connections between obesity, culture, and health.

Right now we are also examining how the distribution and variation of cultural knowledge about obesity within the South Phoenix social network shapes the likelihood of body image distortion and depression and the likelihood of being overweight, including how that pattern differs for men and women. Part of Dressler's theory of cultural consonance (Dressler 1995, 1999, 2004) predicts that failing to understand the norm/ideal is innately and profoundly stressful, as is the inability to reach that norm due to economic or other constraints (see chapter 5 and appendix D). This theory might help explain some of these complex relationships.

Ultimately, questions that seek to explicate the links among the cultural, biological, and ecological contexts of obesity as a complex dynamic will likely be the best way to develop a satisfactory understanding of obesity as a human condition. In particular, we need to understand the complex pathways of obesity across the cultural, biological, and ecological domains of modern human life, so that we can know if, when, and how we should worry about obesity, and ultimately what to do about it.

APPENDIX A. GLOBAL RATES OF OVERWEIGHT AND OBESITY

TABLE A1

Overweight Adults, by Country, 2009

Rank	Country	% Overweight Adults (BMI over 25)
1.	Nauru	94.5
2.	Federated States of Micronesia	91.1
3.	Cook Islands	90.9
4.	Tonga	90.8
5.	Niue	81.7
6.	Samoa	80.4
7.	Palau	78.4
8.	Kuwait	74.2
9.	United States	74.1
10.	Kiribati	73.6
11.	Dominica	71.0
12.	Barbados	69.7
13.	Argentina	69.4
14.	Egypt	69.4
15.	Malta	68.7
16.	Greece	68.5
17.	New Zealand	68.4
18.	United Arab Emirates	68.3
19.	Mexico	68.1
20.	Trinidad and Tobago	67.9
21.	Australia	67.4

(continued)

TABLE A1

Overweight Adults, by Country, 2009 *(continued)*

Rank	Country	% Overweight Adults (BMI over 25)
22.	Belarus	66.8
23.	Chile	65.3
24.	Venezuela	65.2
25.	Seychelles	64.6
26.	Bahrain	64.1
27.	Andorra	63.8
28.	United Kingdom	63.8
29.	Saudi Arabia	63.5
30.	Monaco	62.4
31.	Bolivia	62.2
32.	San Marino	62.1
33.	Guatemala	61.2
34.	Mongolia	61.2
35.	Canada	61.1
36.	Qatar	61.0
37.	Uruguay	60.9
38.	Jordan	60.5
39.	Bahamas	60.4
40.	Iceland	60.4
41.	Nicaragua	60.4
42.	Cuba	60.1
43.	Germany	60.1
44.	Brunei Darussalam	59.8
45.	Slovenia	59.8
46.	Peru	59.6
47.	Vanuatu	59.6
48.	Finland	58.7
49.	Jamaica	57.4
50.	Israel	57.3

(continued)

TABLE AI

Overweight Adults, by Country, 2009 *(continued)*

Rank	Country	% Overweight Adults (BMI over 25)
51.	Saint Lucia	57.3
52.	Austria	57.1
53.	Azerbaijan	57.1
54.	Turkey	56.8
55.	Tuvalu	56.6
56.	Dominican Republic	56.5
57.	Slovakia	56.3
58.	Cyprus	56.2
59.	Saint Kitts and Nevis	56.1
60.	Costa Rica	55.8
61.	Colombia	55.6
62.	Antigua and Barbuda	55.5
63.	Switzerland	55.4
64.	Montenegro	54.9
65.	Serbia	54.9
66.	Serbia and Montenegro	54.9
67.	Albania	54.8
68.	Fiji	54.8
69.	Bulgaria	54.2
70.	Luxembourg	54.2
71.	Croatia	53.9
72.	Bosnia and Herzegovina	53.8
73.	Portugal	53.8
74.	Armenia	53.3
75.	Grenada	53.3
76.	South Africa	53.3
77.	Iran	53.2
78.	Libya	53.2
79.	Lithuania	53.1

(continued)

TABLE A1

Overweight Adults, by Country, 2009 *(continued)*

Rank	Country	% Overweight Adults (BMI over 25)
80.	Lebanon	53.0
81.	Czech Republic	52.9
82.	Syria	52.8
83.	Spain	51.8
84.	Hungary	51.6
85.	Panama	51.4
86.	Tunisia	51.0
87.	Saint Vincent and the Grenadines	50.6
88.	Brazil	50.5
89.	Belize	49.8
90.	Sweden	49.7
91.	Norway	49.1
92.	Russian Federation	49.1
93.	El Salvador	48.7
94.	Lesotho	48.5
95.	Suriname	47.8
96.	Paraguay	47.7
97.	Guyana	47.5
98.	Poland	47.5
99.	Latvia	47.3
100.	Macedonia	47.2
101.	Ecuador	47.1
102.	Turkmenistan	46.8
103.	Ireland	46.6
104.	Belgium	46.3
105.	Marshall Islands	46.2
106.	Netherlands	46.0
107.	Uzbekistan	46.0

(continued)

TABLE A1

Overweight Adults, by Country, 2009 *(continued)*

Rank	Country	% Overweight Adults (BMI over 25)
108.	Denmark	45.8
109.	Mauritius	45.6
110.	Oman	45.6
111.	Italy	45.5
112.	Iraq	45.4
113.	Georgia	44.8
114.	Ukraine	44.8
115.	Solomon Islands	44.0
116.	Botswana	43.6
117.	Honduras	43.5
118.	Equatorial Guinea	43.0
119.	Morocco	42.9
120.	Timor-Leste	42.7
121.	Mauritania	42.5
122.	Estonia	42.2
123.	South Korea	42.0
124.	Swaziland	41.8
125.	Kazakhstan	41.4
126.	Republic of Moldova	41.1
127.	Bhutan	40.9
128.	France	40.1
129.	Cameroon	39.9
130.	Maldives	39.9
131.	Algeria	39.8
132.	North Korea	39.4
133.	Kyrgyzstan	39.2
134.	Romania	39.1
135.	Laos	38.9

(continued)

TABLE A1

Overweight Adults, by Country, 2009 *(continued)*

Rank	Country	*% Overweight Adults (BMI over 25)*
136.	Cape Verde	38.2
137.	Tajikistan	37.3
138.	Gabon	36.5
139.	Myanmar	36.3
140.	Liberia	35.6
141.	Sierra Leone	33.4
142.	Haiti	32.8
143.	Zimbabwe	32.1
144.	Thailand	31.6
145.	Papua New Guinea	30.2
146.	Malaysia	29.9
147.	Ghana	29.2
148.	China	28.9
149.	Benin	28.5
150.	Comoros	28.0
151.	Angola	27.5
152.	Nigeria	27.1
153.	Yemen	27.0
154.	Senegal	26.4
155.	Philippines	25.2
156.	Djibouti	24.9
157.	Mali	24.1
158.	Togo	24.0
159.	Guinea	23.5
160.	Sudan	23.1
161.	Cote d'Ivoire	22.9
162.	Singapore	22.9
163.	Japan	22.6
164.	Namibia	22.5
165.	Pakistan	22.2

(continued)

TABLE A1

Overweight Adults, by Country, 2009 *(continued)*

Rank	Country	% Overweight Adults (BMI over 25)
166.	Sao Tome and Principe	21.4
167.	Tanzania	21.2
168.	Malawi	19.3
169.	Congo, Republic of the	18.9
170.	Niger	17.6
171.	Madagascar	17.4
172.	Mozambique	17.3
173.	Guinea-Bissau	16.7
174.	Gambia	16.6
175.	Indonesia	16.2
176.	India	16.0
177.	Somalia	15.8
178.	Chad	15.6
179.	Afghanistan	15.1
180.	Uganda	14.8
181.	Kenya	14.3
182.	Burkina Faso	14.1
183.	Rwanda	13.7
184.	Zambia	13.0
185.	Burundi	12.9
186.	Central African Republic	12.9
187.	Cambodia	11.3
188.	Congo, Democratic Republic of the	9.1
189.	Nepal	8.4
190.	Sri Lanka	7.4
191.	Viet Nam	6.4
192.	Bangladesh	6.1
193.	Ethiopia	5.6
194.	Eritrea	4.4

Source: From the World Health Organization global database
on BMI, www.who.int/bmi/.

TABLE A2

Mean BMI of Obese and Overweight Adults, by Country and Gender, 2005

	Mean BMI		% Obese (BMI >30)		% Overweight (BMI > 25)	
	Female	Male	Female	Male	Female	Male
Afghanistan	21.5	21.2	1.4	0.5	17.4	12.7
Albania	25.8	26.0	23.8	18.6	52.5	57.2
Algeria	24.6	23.5	13.4	5.2	45.6	34.1
Andorra	27.3	26.2	28.8	15.8	66.8	60.9
Angola	23.2	22.1	6.9	1.9	33.6	21.3
Antigua and Barbuda	26.4	25.2	22.9	11.2	59.8	51.2
Argentina	27.5	27.9	31.0	31.4	65.7	73.1
Armenia	25.7	25.5	19.8	12.1	52.8	53.9
Australia	26.8	27.3	24.9	23.8	62.7	72.1
Austria	25.9	26.5	20.3	21.3	53.2	61.0
Azerbaijan	26.4	25.9	24.9	15.4	56.8	57.4
Bahamas	26.9	25.8	27.1	14.7	63.8	57.0
Bahrain	27.9	26.4	35.2	21.2	67.3	60.9
Bangladesh	19.6	20.2	0.2	0.1	5.4	6.7
Barbados	30.3	26.1	50.8	16.8	80.1	59.2
Belarus	27.7	26.3	32.2	16.2	69.9	63.7
Belgium	24.2	25.4	9.5	13.3	40.7	51.9
Belize	25.7	24.6	18.6	7.9	54.9	44.7
Benin	23.8	21.9	9.3	1.0	39.1	17.9
Bhutan	24.7	23.6	14.3	5.8	46.5	35.3
Bolivia	27.7	25.8	33.1	14.7	68.0	56.3
Bosnia and Herzegovina	25.7	25.8	21.5	13.8	51.0	56.6
Botswana	25.1	23.9	14.6	5.4	49.4	37.8
Brazil	25.6	24.8	18.3	8.7	53.5	47.4
Brunei Darussalam	26.9	25.8	27.4	15.2	63.2	56.4
Bulgaria	25.0	26.3	19.0	17.0	45.5	62.8

(continued)

TABLE A2

**Mean BMI of Obese and Overweight Adults,
by Country and Gender, 2005** *(continued)*

	Mean BMI		*% Obese (BMI >30)*		*% Overweight (BMI > 25)*	
	Female	*Male*	*Female*	*Male*	*Female*	*Male*
Burkina Faso	21.3	21.2	1.1	0.4	16.0	12.1
Burundi	21.7	20.5	1.5	0.1	18.1	7.8
Cambodia	21.2	22.1	0.1	0.2	9.3	13.3
Cameroon	24.1	24.0	10.8	7.5	41.1	38.7
Canada	26.1	26.8	23.2	23.7	57.1	65.1
Cape Verde	24.4	23.3	12.5	4.6	44.1	32.4
Central African Republic	21.9	20.9	1.3	0.1	18.5	7.2
Chad	21.7	21.2	1.7	0.4	19.2	12.0
Chile	27.6	26.4	31.6	19.0	68.0	62.6
China	22.8	23.7	1.9	1.6	24.7	33.1
Colombia	25.8	25.8	19.9	14.9	54.6	56.5
Comoros	23.5	22.1	7.1	1.2	35.9	20.0
Congo, Democratic Republic of the	21.1	19.9	0.8	0.0	13.3	4.8
Congo, Republic of the	22.5	21.4	3.0	0.4	25.2	12.7
Cook Islands	34.0	32.8	70.8	69.5	89.2	92.6
Costa Rica	26.4	25.5	24.2	13.0	57.8	53.9
Cote d'Ivoire	23.4	21.5	5.4	0.2	34.2	11.6
Croatia	25.0	26.3	16.2	18.2	46.4	61.3
Cuba	26.6	26.0	24.6	14.9	61.1	59.2
Cyprus	26.4	25.3	22.2	10.1	60.6	51.7
Czech Republic	25.3	26.1	20.7	18.5	47.8	58.1
Denmark	24.0	25.3	7.1	10.6	39.1	52.5
Djibouti	22.9	21.8	5.8	1.4	31.0	18.9
Dominica	29.6	26.6	46.0	20.0	77.1	65.1
Dominican Republic	27.5	24.8	31.8	7.7	66.4	46.6
Ecuador	25.4	24.3	16.7	6.7	52.6	41.7

(continued)

TABLE A2

**Mean BMI of Obese and Overweight Adults,
by Country and Gender, 2005** *(continued)*

	Mean BMI		% Obese (BMI >30)		% Overweight (BMI > 25)	
	Female	*Male*	*Female*	*Male*	*Female*	*Male*
Egypt	29.6	26.7	45.5	22.0	74.2	64.5
El Salvador	25.6	24.5	17.8	7.4	54.0	43.5
Equatorial Guinea	24.9	23.8	15.4	6.4	48.5	37.5
Eritrea	20.2	20.0	0.1	0.0	5.7	3.1
Estonia	23.5	25.1	8.4	8.6	33.8	50.7
Ethiopia	19.8	20.6	0.0	0.2	3.3	7.8
Fiji	27.6	24.5	32.5	8.7	65.6	43.9
Finland	25.6	26.6	17.8	18.9	52.4	64.9
France	23.7	24.7	6.6	7.8	34.7	45.6
Gabon	24.9	22.6	15.5	2.3	47.7	25.4
Gambia	22.1	20.8	2.5	0.3	22.8	10.3
Georgia	25.2	24.1	14.7	5.2	50.8	38.9
Germany	26.0	26.7	20.4	20.9	55.1	65.1
Ghana	22.6	23.1	4.2	3.3	28.1	30.3
Greece	26.7	27.7	24.5	27.7	61.3	75.7
Grenada	26.1	25.0	21.2	9.8	58.0	48.7
Guatemala	27.3	25.9	29.7	15.7	65.4	56.9
Guinea	22.9	21.7	5.2	0.8	30.4	16.5
Guinea-Bissau	21.9	20.8	2.8	0.5	22.1	11.4
Guyana	25.5	24.4	17.0	6.8	52.9	42.1
Haiti	25.2	21.6	15.0	0.7	50.6	15.1
Honduras	25.1	23.9	14.4	5.2	49.4	37.6
Hungary	25.1	25.8	16.1	15.8	47.4	55.9
Iceland	26.6	26.1	23.2	16.7	61.7	59.0
India	21.1	21.6	1.4	1.1	15.2	16.8
Indonesia	22.2	21.0	2.6	0.2	22.7	9.7
Iran	26.5	24.9	27.0	10.0	57.8	48.5

(continued)

TABLE A2

Mean BMI of Obese and Overweight Adults,
by Country and Gender, 2005 *(continued)*

| | Mean BMI | | % Obese (BMI >30) | | % Overweight (BMI > 25) | |
	Female	Male	Female	Male	Female	Male
Iraq	25.2	24.1	16.8	7.2	50.8	40.1
Ireland	24.3	25.3	9.1	10.3	41.7	51.5
Israel	26.5	25.9	24.3	16.2	57.5	57.2
Italy	24.2	25.5	12.6	12.9	38.3	52.7
Jamaica	28.8	24.2	41.0	5.1	74.7	40.0
Japan	21.9	23.1	1.5	1.8	18.1	27.0
Jordan	27.9	26.1	35.6	19.6	63.4	57.5
Kazakhstan	24.0	24.6	11.0	7.9	38.9	43.9
Kenya	22.2	20.6	1.9	0.1	21.7	6.9
Kiribati	28.8	27.8	41.0	29.8	73.9	73.2
Kuwait	31.0	27.5	52.9	29.6	79.0	69.5
Kyrgyzstan	24.7	23.6	14.2	5.0	43.9	34.5
Laos	24.7	23.6	10.4	2.6	45.6	32.1
Latvia	24.8	25.1	15.0	9.7	44.7	49.9
Lebanon	26.2	25.3	25.2	14.9	54.3	51.7
Lesotho	27.9	23.1	34.3	1.9	69.5	27.5
Liberia	24.1	23.0	11.0	3.8	41.6	29.6
Libya	26.1	25.0	22.5	11.4	57.5	48.8
Lithuania	24.7	26.3	13.9	16.8	43.9	62.3
Luxembourg	25.6	25.6	16.0	12.1	54.0	54.4
Macedonia	26.4	23.9	24.3	5.9	57.4	37.1
Madagascar	21.8	21.1	1.9	1.0	20.2	14.5
Malawi	22.4	21.7	2.0	0.7	23.5	15.1
Malaysia	23.7	22.5	8.2	1.6	37.2	22.7
Maldives	25.3	23.2	22.0	5.7	47.6	32.3
Mali	23.2	21.5	6.2	0.6	33.6	14.6
Malta	28.1	27.4	34.8	25.9	66.1	71.4
Marshall Islands	25.3	24.2	16.1	6.3	51.8	40.6

(continued)

TABLE A2

**Mean BMI of Obese and Overweight Adults,
by Country and Gender, 2005** *(continued)*

	Mean BMI		% Obese (BMI >30)		% Overweight (BMI > 25)	
	Female	*Male*	*Female*	*Male*	*Female*	*Male*
Mauritania	25.9	23.1	22.9	3.7	54.6	30.4
Mauritius	25.4	24.0	18.3	5.6	52.3	39.0
Mexico	27.9	27.1	34.3	24.0	67.9	68.4
Micronesia, Federated States of	34.7	32.2	72.9	66.2	90.1	92.1
Moldova	24.9	23.7	12.5	4.0	47.4	34.8
Monaco	27.1	26.0	27.5	14.5	65.6	59.1
Mongolia	27.4	25.3	29.0	7.9	69.3	53.0
Montenegro	25.4	26.3	20.6	17.7	48.5	61.2
Morocco	25.8	23.2	20.5	3.7	54.7	31.1
Mozambique	22.5	21.1	3.0	0.2	25.3	9.3
Myanmar	24.5	23.3	9.1	2.1	43.3	29.4
Namibia	23.2	21.5	5.3	0.3	32.6	12.3
Nauru	36.5	35.8	78.8	83.2	92.4	96.5
Nepal	20.3	20.7	0.2	0.2	8.0	8.8
Netherlands	24.6	25.0	11.5	10.4	44.0	48.0
New Zealand	27.6	27.1	31.5	23.0	68.2	68.7
Nicaragua	27.9	25.4	34.3	11.5	68.1	52.9
Niger	21.9	21.4	2.3	0.6	21.3	13.9
Nigeria	23.1	22.2	6.0	2.0	32.2	21.9
Niue	32.1	28.6	61.0	36.8	85.0	78.5
North Korea	24.8	23.6	10.7	2.7	46.2	32.7
Norway	24.4	25.5	9.3	11.3	43.4	54.8
Oman	24.9	24.4	14.8	7.7	47.8	43.4
Pakistan	22.3	22.0	3.6	1.0	25.5	18.8
Palau	30.9	28.0	55.0	31.2	82.4	74.5
Panama	25.9	24.8	19.8	8.8	56.3	46.5

(continued)

TABLE A2

**Mean BMI of Obese and Overweight Adults,
by Country and Gender, 2005** *(continued)*

	Mean BMI		% Obese (BMI >30)		% Overweight (BMI > 25)	
	Female	*Male*	*Female*	*Male*	*Female*	*Male*
Papua New Guinea	22.9	23.4	4.2	2.5	29.0	31.5
Paraguay	25.5	24.4	17.2	7.0	53.2	42.3
Peru	27.4	25.6	31.1	13.2	64.7	54.6
Philippines	22.8	22.5	3.7	1.1	28.5	21.9
Poland	24.8	25.3	18.0	12.9	44.3	50.7
Portugal	25.2	25.9	16.1	13.7	49.2	58.5
Qatar	27.1	26.0	29.3	17.4	64.1	57.9
Romania	24.2	23.9	12.0	5.5	40.6	37.7
Russian Federation	25.9	24.9	23.6	9.6	51.7	46.5
Rwanda	22.1	20.9	1.3	0.1	20.1	7.3
Saint Kitts and Nevis	26.4	25.3	23.4	11.6	60.3	52.0
Saint Lucia	27.9	24.6	34.7	6.6	69.1	45.5
Saint Vincent and the Grenadines	25.8	24.7	19.2	8.4	55.7	45.6
Samoa	31.8	28.8	57.3	38.4	82.1	78.7
San Marino	27.1	25.9	27.2	14.3	65.4	58.8
Sao Tome and Principe	22.5	21.4	4.4	0.9	27.2	15.5
Saudi Arabia	27.6	26.6	33.8	23.0	63.8	63.1
Senegal	23.6	21.2	9.2	1.3	36.7	16.1
Serbia	25.4	26.3	20.6	17.7	48.5	61.2
Serbia and Montenegro	25.4	26.3	20.6	17.7	48.5	61.2
Seychelles	28.4	25.9	38.6	16.7	70.7	58.5
Sierra Leone	24.5	22.1	12.7	2.4	44.5	22.4
Singapore	22.2	22.7	1.8	1.3	22.0	23.8
Slovakia	26.4	25.3	22.8	10.8	60.6	52.0
Slovenia	26.8	25.7	25.2	12.5	63.5	56.0
Solomon Islands	25.1	24.0	14.7	5.4	49.9	38.2

(continued)

TABLE A2

**Mean BMI of Obese and Overweight Adults,
by Country and Gender, 2005** *(continued)*

	Mean BMI		% Obese (BMI >30)		% Overweight (BMI > 25)	
	Female	*Male*	*Female*	*Male*	*Female*	*Male*
Somalia	21.8	20.7	2.6	0.4	21.1	10.6
South Africa	27.9	24.1	35.2	6.7	67.2	39.3
South Korea	24.6	24.3	10.1	4.1	43.8	40.2
Spain	25.2	25.8	15.8	15.6	47.7	55.8
Sri Lanka	20.2	20.9	0.1	0.2	5.9	8.9
Sudan	22.7	21.6	5.1	1.2	29.1	17.2
Suriname	25.5	24.4	17.2	7.0	53.2	42.4
Swaziland	24.9	23.8	13.5	4.7	47.8	35.8
Sweden	24.6	25.5	10.9	11.8	44.9	54.5
Switzerland	25.9	25.6	18.7	12.4	56.7	54.1
Syrian Arab Republic	26.1	24.9	22.2	11.2	57.2	48.4
Tajikistan	24.5	23.4	10.4	2.9	43.9	30.8
Tanzania	22.7	21.8	3.1	0.7	27.0	15.4
Thailand	23.5	23.0	8.4	2.5	35.2	27.9
Timor-Leste	24.9	23.8	15.4	6.5	48.2	37.2
Togo	23.0	21.8	5.3	0.9	30.9	17.1
Tonga	35.7	31.4	76.1	60.7	91.4	90.3
Trinidad and Tobago	29.6	25.9	46.1	14.0	77.0	58.9
Tunisia	26.9	24.4	30.2	7.7	59.2	42.8
Turkey	27.6	25.0	32.5	10.8	65.7	47.9
Turkmenistan	24.9	25.0	15.0	9.3	45.5	48.1
Tuvalu	26.5	25.3	23.8	11.9	60.7	52.5
Uganda	22.3	20.9	1.6	0.1	22.2	7.4
Ukraine	25.4	24.3	19.4	7.4	48.5	41.2
United Arab Emirates	28.6	27.0	39.4	24.5	69.6	66.9
United Kingdom	26.7	26.8	24.2	21.6	61.9	65.7

(continued)

TABLE A2

Mean BMI of Obese and Overweight Adults, by Country and Gender, 2005 *(continued)*

	Mean BMI		% Obese (BMI >30)		% Overweight (BMI > 25)	
	Female	*Male*	*Female*	*Male*	*Female*	*Male*
United States	28.8	28.4	41.8	36.5	72.6	75.6
Uruguay	26.3	26.6	23.3	20.1	58.1	63.6
Uzbekistan	25.4	24.4	17.6	7.1	49.9	42.0
Vanuatu	26.8	25.7	26.3	13.4	62.9	56.3
Venezuela	26.7	27.0	26.2	23.2	61.4	69.1
Viet Nam	20.6	20.8	0.3	0.0	8.7	4.1
Yemen	22.8	22.6	5.1	2.0	29.4	24.6
Zambia	21.9	20.9	1.3	0.1	18.6	7.5
Zimbabwe	25.1	21.8	15.3	0.6	48.9	15.3

Sources: Adapted from Ono, Guthold, and Strong 2005 and the World Health Organization global BMI database (www.who.int/bmi/).

APPENDIX B. BODY MASS INDEX TABLES

TABLE B1
BMI Estimator for Adults

BMI	19	20	21	22	23	24	25	26	27	28	29	30	31	32	33	34	35
Height (inches)								Body Weight (pounds)									
58	91	96	100	105	110	115	119	124	129	134	138	143	148	153	158	162	167
59	94	99	104	109	114	119	124	128	133	138	143	148	153	158	163	168	173
60	97	102	107	112	118	123	128	133	138	143	148	153	158	163	168	174	179
61	100	106	111	116	122	127	132	137	143	148	153	158	164	169	174	180	185
62	104	109	115	120	126	131	136	142	147	153	158	164	169	175	180	186	191
63	107	113	118	124	130	135	141	146	152	158	163	169	175	180	186	191	197
64	110	116	122	128	134	140	145	151	157	163	169	174	180	186	192	197	204
65	114	120	126	132	138	144	150	156	162	168	174	180	186	192	198	204	210
66	118	124	130	136	142	148	155	161	167	173	179	186	192	198	204	210	216
67	121	127	134	140	146	153	159	166	172	178	185	191	198	204	211	217	223
68	125	131	138	144	151	158	164	171	177	184	190	197	203	210	216	223	230
69	128	135	142	149	155	162	169	176	182	189	196	203	209	216	223	230	236
70	132	139	146	153	160	167	174	181	188	195	202	209	216	222	229	236	243
71	136	143	150	157	165	172	179	186	193	200	208	215	222	229	236	243	250
72	140	147	154	162	169	177	184	191	199	206	213	221	228	235	242	250	258
73	144	151	159	166	174	182	189	197	204	212	219	227	235	242	250	257	265
74	148	155	163	171	179	186	194	202	210	218	225	233	241	249	256	264	272
75	152	160	168	176	184	192	200	208	216	224	232	240	248	256	264	272	279
76	156	164	172	180	189	197	205	213	221	230	238	246	254	263	271	279	287

BMI											Body Weight (pounds)								
Height (inches)	36	37	38	39	40	41	42	43	44	45	46	47	48	49	50	51	52	53	54
58	172	177	181	186	191	196	201	205	210	215	220	224	229	234	239	244	248	253	258
59	178	183	188	193	198	203	208	212	217	222	227	232	237	242	247	252	257	262	267
60	184	189	194	199	204	209	215	220	225	230	235	240	245	250	255	261	266	271	276
61	190	195	201	206	211	217	222	227	232	238	243	248	254	259	264	269	275	280	285
62	196	202	207	213	218	224	229	235	240	246	251	256	262	267	273	278	284	289	295
63	203	208	214	220	225	231	237	242	248	254	259	265	270	278	282	287	293	299	304
64	209	215	221	227	232	238	244	250	256	262	267	273	279	285	291	296	302	308	314
65	216	222	228	234	240	246	252	258	264	270	276	282	288	294	300	306	312	318	324
66	223	229	235	241	247	253	260	266	272	278	284	291	297	303	309	315	322	328	334
67	230	236	242	249	255	261	268	274	280	287	293	299	306	312	319	325	331	338	344
68	236	243	249	256	262	269	276	282	289	295	302	308	315	322	328	335	341	348	354
69	243	250	257	263	270	277	284	291	297	304	311	318	324	331	338	345	351	358	365
70	250	257	264	271	278	285	292	299	306	313	320	327	334	341	348	355	362	369	376
71	257	265	272	279	286	293	301	308	315	322	329	338	343	351	358	365	372	379	386
72	265	272	279	287	294	302	309	316	324	331	338	346	353	361	368	375	383	390	397
73	272	280	288	295	302	310	318	325	333	340	348	355	363	371	378	386	393	401	408
74	280	287	295	303	311	319	326	334	342	350	358	365	373	381	389	396	404	412	420
75	287	295	303	311	319	327	335	343	351	359	367	375	383	391	399	407	415	423	431
76	295	304	312	320	328	336	344	353	361	369	377	385	394	402	410	418	426	435	443

Note: To estimate BMI, find the cell that matches body weight (in pounds) on the line that matches height (in inches). The corresponding figure in the top row is the estimated BMI. (Pounds have been rounded.)

TABLE B2

Standard International BMI Cutoff Points for Defining
Overweight and Obesity in Children

Age (years)	Minimum BMI Categorized as Overweight[a]		Minimum BMI Categorized as Obese[b]	
	Male	Female	Male	Female
2	18.41	18.02	20.09	19.81
2.5	18.13	17.76	19.80	19.55
3	17.89	17.56	19.57	19.36
3.5	17.69	17.40	19.39	19.23
4	17.55	17.28	19.29	19.15
4.5	17.47	17.19	19.26	19.12
5	17.42	17.15	19.30	19.17
5.5	17.45	17.20	19.47	19.34
6	17.55	17.34	19.78	19.65
6.5	17.71	17.53	20.23	20.08
7	17.92	17.75	20.63	20.51
7.5	18.16	18.03	21.09	21.01
8	18.44	18.35	21.60	21.57
8.5	18.76	18.69	22.17	22.18
9	19.10	19.07	22.77	22.81
9.5	19.46	19.45	23.39	23.46
10	19.84	19.86	24.00	24.11
10.5	20.20	20.29	24.57	24.77
11	20.55	20.74	25.10	25.42
11.5	20.89	21.20	25.58	26.05
12	21.22	21.68	26.02	26.67
12.5	21.56	22.14	26.43	27.24
13	21.91	22.58	26.84	27.76
13.5	22.27	22.98	27.25	28.20
14	22.62	23.34	27.63	28.57
14.5	22.96	23.66	27.98	28.87
15	23.29	23.94	28.30	29.11
15.5	23.60	24.17	28.60	29.29
16	23.90	24.37	28.88	29.43
16.5	24.19	24.54	29.14	29.56
17	24.46	24.70	29.41	29.69
17.5	24.73	24.85	29.70	29.84
18	25	25	30	30

Source: From Cole et al. 2000.
[a]Comparable to adult BMI of 25 kg/m^2
[b]Comparable to adult BMI of 30 kg/m^2

APPENDIX C. TOOLS FOR THE
COMPARATIVE STUDY OF BODY IMAGE

The body image studies discussed in chapter 5 use a range of different scales to measure people's perceptions of their current and ideal sizes. Most commonly, respondents are presented with a series of pictures of standardized bodies of scaled sizes and asked which one best approximates their current size and which one they would most like to be. The scales come in different forms: figural drawings, silhouettes, manipulated photographs, and computerized images that respondents can adjust. The Figure Rating Scale (FRS) described in Stunkard, Sorensen, and Schulsinger 1983, and shown in the figure, is a nine-figure line-drawing scale as valid and reliable as newer more technologically sophisticated versions of body image scales. The FRS has been used as an ordinal scale but is most often used as an interval one (Demarest and Allen 2000; Perry, Rosenblatt, and Wang 2004). It is probably the most widely used, and for investigative studies in cross-cultural settings, the one I recommend. It is simple but it seems to work (Bulik et al. 2005), and is easy to adapt. Comparative results from a range of previous studies using this tool or its adaptations are given in the table. Our Samoan study used figures rendered to have recognizably Samoan body proportions and hairstyle.

BMIs are also attached to each figure (see Stunkard 2000) and given in the table following, and Rand and Wright (2000) provide a matched scale of nine figures representing children's bodies. Another scale used in a number of cross-cultural body image studies is the twelve-figure scale of Furnham and Alibhai (1983). The BIA silhouette scale, developed specifically for use with women with eating disorders, now includes (as the BIA-O) very obese bodies (Williamson et al. 2000) and gives some of the best differentiation at the upper end of the scale. Thompson (1996) reviews forty-two methods of body image assessment for those wanting to explore the fullest range of options.

Fingeret, Gleaves, and Pearson (2004) provide a basic discussion of the assumptions to be considered in selecting the right scale(s) for a body image study. Some scales apply only to women; others include men or children. I recommend using an established scale, even if it needs slight modification for a specific study. Most scales were originally presented as a series of graduated body sizes ordered from small to large, although more recently there is some discussion that it might be better to present the bodies in some randomly arranged order (Fingeret, Gleaves, and Pearson 2004). I have found that line drawings rather than photos or computer-based tools work best in diverse cross-cultural settings, because they tend to be the most comfortable for people who might not have great familiarity with photographs or computers; for example, when we pretested several potential body image measurement tools with Samoans, including photographic and computer-generated images, participants more easily distinguished and managed line drawings. In South Phoenix, where people are more accustomed to computer and photographic images, we have found photo-based scales work better.

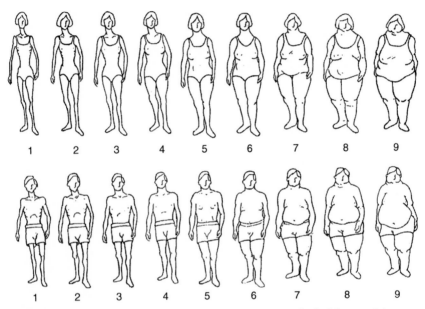

FIGURE C1 The Figural Rating Scale (Stunkard, Sorensen, and Schulsinger 1983).

TABLE CI

Samples of Women's Mean BMI and Responses to the Stunkard Figural Rating Scale (FRS)

			Body Size on 1–9 FRS (Mean)		
	Sample size	Mean BMI	Size They Rate Themselves To Be	Size They Would Like To Be	Source
University Students (or Similarly Aged and Educated) Samples					
University of Pennsylvania psychology students					Rozin, Trachtenberg, and Cohen 2001
1983–1984	200	20	3.5	2.8	
1995–1998	302	21	3.5	2.8	
U.S. university students	83	23	4.9	3.1	Forbes et al. 2005
U.S. university students	166	N/A	N/A	3.3	Rand and Wright 2000
U.S. undergraduate psychology students	34	22	3.4	2.5	Lamb et al. 1993
Young women of Iranian descent, Los Angeles	45	21	3.5	2.8	Abdollahi and Mann 2001
New Zealand university students	119	24	4.4	3.2	Miller and Halbertstadt 2005
Australian university students	149	22	4.2	2.8	Mahmud and Crittenden 2007
Australian university students	275	22	4.7	3.3	Tiggemann and Ruutel 2001
Estonian university students	258	21	3.8	3.1	Tiggemann and Ruutel 2001
Polish university students	111	20	3.7	3.0	Forbes et al. 2004
Pakistani university students	278	21	3.3	2.6	Mahmud and Crittenden 2007

(continued)

TABLE C1

Samples of Women's Mean BMI and Responses to the Stunkard Figural Rating Scale (FRS) *(continued)*

	Sample size	Mean BMI	*Body Size on 1–9 FRS* *(Mean)*		Source
			Size They Rate Themselves To Be	*Size They Would Like To Be*	
Israeli university students (Arab and Jewish)	96	20	3.3	3.0	Safir, Flaisher-Kellner, and Rosenmann 2005
Taiwanese university students	165	21	3.5	2.8	Shih and Kubo 2002
Portuguese university students	98	22	3.5	2.8	Scagliusi et al. 2006
Thai university-age students	24	N/A	N/A	2.9	Sharps, Sharps-Price, and Hanson 2001
Tehran university students	59	22	3.5	2.8	Abdollahi and Mann 2001
Adult Samples					
U.S., over 40 years	42	25	4.3	2.6	Lamb et al. 1993
U.S., middle-aged	205	N/A	N/A	3.8	Rand and Wright 2000
White Virginians, 18–100 years	16728	24	4.1	3.2	Bulik et al. 2001
U.S., Asian	189	21	3.4	2.7	Cachelin et al. 2002
U.S., Black	132	27	4.1	3.1	Cachelin et al. 2002
U.S., Hispanic	379	25	3.9	2.9	Cachelin et al. 2002
U.S., White	101	23	3.7	2.7	Cachelin et al. 2002

(continued)

TABLE CI

Samples of Women's Mean BMI and Responses to the Stunkard Figural Rating Scale (FRS) (continued)

	Sample size	Mean BMI	Body Size on 1–9 FRS (Mean)		Source
			Size They Rate Themselves To Be	Size They Would Like To Be	
Chicago, Latin American primary caregivers of young children	234	31	4.6	3.5	Sanchez-Johnsen et al. 2004
Chicago, Black primary caregivers of young children	271	30	5.0	3.1	Sanchez-Johnsen et al.2004
Ontario, Ojibway-Cree	426	27	4.6	3.7	Gittelsohn et al. 1996
Australia, suburban, 18–59 years	180	N/A	4.0	3.3	Stevens and Tiggemann 1998
Netherlands, Turkish	122	25.6	4.3	3.4	Nicolau et al. 2008
Netherlands, Moroccan	104	24.1	4.6	3.9	Nicolau et al. 2008
Ukraine, urban, 18–60 years	616	22	3.2	2.7	Bilukha and Utermohlen 2002
Samoa	84	31	3.7	2.9	Brewis and McGarvey 2000; Brewis et al. 1998
American Samoa	76	36	4.8	3.5	Brewis and McGarvey 2000, Brewis et al. 1998
Samoans in Auckland, New Zealand	41	34	4.5	2.4	Brewis and McGarvey 2000; Brewis et al. 1998

(continued)

TABLE C1

Samples of Women's Mean BMI and Responses to the Stunkard Figural Rating Scale (FRS) *(continued)*

	Sample size	Mean BMI	Body Size on 1–9 FRS (Mean)		Source
			Size They Rate Themselves To Be	*Size They Would Like To Be*	
High school teachers, Japan	45	N/A	N/A	3.5	Smith and Joiner 2008
Qatar, Arab	535	N/A	N/A	3.4	Musaiger, Shahbeek, and Al-Mannai 2004
Younger Samples					
Virginia, young rural adolescents					Jones, Fries, and Danish 2007
Black	219	22	3.7	3.5	
White	165	20	3.2	2.9	
Mexico, public school girls, 12–15 years, from a small city	137	N/A	3.7	3.0	Austin and Smith 2008

Note: Where no location is listed for a sample, the location was unspecified.

TABLE C2

Estimated BMIs for the Nine Figural Rating Scale Body Figures

	Figure Number								
	1	2	3	4	5	6	7	8	9
Women	18.3	19.3	20.9	23.1	26.2	29.9	34.3	38.6	45.4
Men	19.8	21.1	22.2	23.6	25.8	28.1	31.5	35.2	41.5

Source: Stunkard, Sorensen, and Schulsinger 1983.
Note: Values are rounded.

APPENDIX D. USING CULTURAL CONSENSUS ANALYSIS TO UNDERSTAND OBESITY NORMS

Cultural consensus analysis (CCA) provides a way to understand empirically how people collectively and differently conceptualize the world around them, including how they think about and understand obesity and big bodies. It is the most commonly applied mathematical description of culture and cultural variation, but it is yet to be applied widely to understanding obesity or the related domains of food, exercise, or body image. Cultural consensus draws on cognitive theories of culture, which emphasize the idea that culture is what is in our heads, that is, the bits of cultural knowledge we get from and give to others and hence share. By eliciting that information in a systematic manner, cultural consensus analysis provides a replicable and comparative means to describe cultural knowledge within specific domains in ways that can then be modeled along with other types of information. For example, it allows us to identify how various cultural ideas about big bodies and obesity are distributed within and across different populations, and to link those to such factors as SES, neighborhood characteristics, or individual body size. It is a method with considerable untapped potential to better explore how cultural understandings about obesity are distributed in a way that could be related systematically to a wide range of other factors, such as actual body size, socioeconomic status, or neighborhood characteristics. It is very good for identifying the cultural source materials from which people draw their beliefs, and for identifying a shared cultural model (Hruschka et al. 2008).

The CCA approach can be used in a wide array of ways to understand culture-obesity connections, because they articulate with both biology and the environments in which we live. We can determine if men and women have different answer keys and if those who are obese do, and how cultural competency varies by such factors as education. In our research in rural Georgia, we used the CCA approach to test if mothers of young children had a shared model relating to healthy ways to feed young children (Brewis and Gartin 2006). Dressler and colleagues (2008) used the approach to test if anthropometric measurements were predicted by people's cultural competency scores related to cultural knowledge about lifestyle aspirations and prestige food (based on freelisting, a different ethnographic technique to elicit the items for analysis). They found those with the highest scores had lower waist measurements and BMIs, and they suggest (an as yet untested proposition) that low cultural consonance in general domains is fundamentally stressful and might lead to greater eating as a stress relief mechanism. Consonance refers to the fit between norms and individual abilities to live up to those norms (i.e., to be slim in a slim-preferring context). In the case of obesity, low consonance would be an anti-fat cultural model paired with a high BMI.

For those interested in using cultural consensus models (CCM), the best references to start with are Weller 2007 and Hrushcka et al. 2008; much of what follows here draws from these two sources. There are several different things you can determine using this approach. These include whether there is a shared cultural model (i.e., consensus in a domain of knowledge) evident in a sample of respondents; whether different groups within a sample (e.g., men and women, the overweight and the normal weight, or those from different countries) are drawing on different cultural models; and which cultural items (beliefs) are most influential in any shared cultural model. Thus, in relation to obesity you can test the degree to which people's shared understandings emphasize individual versus structural explanations for obesity, and which specific beliefs about obesity appear to be most widely held. The analysis can also ascribe a cultural consensus score to an individual within a sample, which indicates how well that person's statements mesh with those of the group. Someone with high consensus scores (say, 0.8) is someone who knows the culturally correct answers most of the time, that is, the individual tends to think what most people think. Some of the advantages of this approach include the ability to use convenience samples if necessary and relatively small samples (ideally, more than forty-five individuals, but with samples of twenty-five it is still possible to run an analysis).

The method starts with a survey tool that includes a series of "cultural statements" posed as either true/false statements or yes/no questions, or with scaled responses. There are a number of different ways the cultural statements can be generated—both inductive and deductive. We used both indicative and deductive means to select our cultural statements about obesity, starting with statements taken from the transcripts of open-ended (qualitative) interviews about people's perceptions of obesity and eating, conducted in a variety of places, including Georgia and Phoenix, in both Spanish and English. We used a text management program to search for key terms and to identify statements made by participants that had the qualities of cultural statements. We then added some statements suggested by the core findings of published ethnographies discussing big bodies and obesity (e.g., "Fat is prestigious," from Sobo's Jamaican study) and my own ethnographic work in Mexico and Samoa. We then added some statements that people hadn't made in interviews, but that are clearly suggested in the public health literature, such as, "Living close to parks or green spaces helps you stay fit and slim." We started with some 100 items and removed all those that people did not respond well to or understand clearly when we did pretesting. We then also removed any duplicative items and reversed some items to reduce response bias. The final list of statements we used is shown in table D1.

The CCM has three basic assumptions shaping survey-tool design: there is a single culturally correct way to respond to a cultural question (a "common truth"); each person's responses are independent of each other; and everyone understands the questions in the same way. For this last reason, selecting simple, clear cultural ideas is critical to good model development. Because the method requires questions to be understood equally well by all respondents, pretesting and care with translation and back translation are very important.

To run a formal consensus analysis, UCINET is the program most often used, but you can also use ANTHROPAC. Both can be purchased online at www.analytictech.com. However, it is also possible to run an informal consensus analysis using standard statistical packages such as SPSS, which may be sufficient for most obesity researchers wishing to do a very rudimentary cultural consensus. The shared cultural model is extracted using factor analysis procedures, with the factors being the respondents rather than the variables (i.e., columns and rows in the dataset are reversed from the usual layout). The first principal component represents the shared cultural model (as long as all the loadings are positive and the ratio between the eigenvalue of the first and second component is greater than 3). The cultural competency scores for individuals are the factor loadings, and should mostly be between 0.5 and 0.8 in a shared model. When we run this factor analysis for individuals, we can identify the shared (consensus) model, that is, the set of culturally correct answers that most people agree on. Generally, the most frequent answer to each statement can be considered the culturally correct answer. To simplify the explanation of the approach, we can examine the "cultural answer key" generated for the group of global health undergraduates from Arizona State University (table D1; second column from the left). By "culturally correct answer," we mean the answer that most people agree on (which may not be scientifically correct, for example).

In some cases, there can be more than one cultural model (more than one set of structured knowledge in a coherent domain [Hrushcka et al. 2008]) that people are influenced by or contributing to, and models may change across populations, for example, with age, cohorts, or across subcultures, or between, say, medical specialists and their patients. For example, we might expect that men's models differ from women's about the consequences of obesity in some key ways, or that Americans and Puerto Ricans draw on a different set of core ideas ("cultural models"). Using competency scores allows us to do some other interesting analyses, such as testing if those with high BMIs tend to be most normative in how they think about obesity.

For our study, we collected data through in-person survey interviews in American Samoa and Tanzania, and with adults in Northern Mexico in the

TABLE D1

Results of a Cross-Cultural Survey and Consensus Analysis of Opinions on Obesity, 2009

	Argentina	ASU	London	New Zealand	Tanzania	Puerto Rico	Paraguay	North Phoenix	Nogales	Samoa	Iceland	All samples
OBESITY IS AN INDIVIDUAL RESPONSIBILITY, AND BASED ON INDIVIDUAL BEHAVIOR												
People who are overweight are the ones that don't like exercising	F	F	F	F	F	F	T	F	T	T	F	F
People are overweight because they are lazy	F	F	F	F	F	F	T	F	T	F	F	F
There isn't much you can do to stop from getting overweight	F	F	F	F	F	F	F	F	F	F	F	F
Some people are just fated to be obese	T	F	F	F	T	F	T	F	T	T	F	F
The best way to lose weight is by exercising	T	T	T	T	T	T	T	T	T	T	T	T
It's important to exercise every day	T	T	T	T	T	T	T	T	T	T	T	T
You need to watch what you eat carefully	T	T	T	T	T	T	T	T	T	T	T	T
Exercising is the best	T	T	T	T	T	T	T	T	T	T	T	T

way to control your weight												
If kids are overweight, the parents are to blame	T	T	T	T	F	T	T	T	T	T	T	T	T
It is important to know how much you weigh	T	T	T	F	T	T	T	T	T	T	T	T	T
You need to be careful about weight gain when you are pregnant	T	T	T	T	T	T	T	T	T	T	T	T	T
Eating high-fat foods in what makes you gain weight	T	T	T	T	T	T	T	T	T	T	T	T	T
If you don't exercise enough you will become overweight	50/50	T	T	T	T	T	T	F	T	T	T	F	T
You need to always watch what you eat so you don't get fat	T	T	T	T	T	T	T	50/50	T	T	T	T	T
Obesity happens when people don't have self control	T	T	T	F	T	T	F	F	T	T	T	T	T
Maintaining an attractive body takes a lot of hard work	T	T	T	T	T	T	T	T	T	T	T	T	T

(continued)

TABLE D1

Results of a Cross-Cultural Survey and Consensus Analysis of Opinions on Obesity, 2009 (continued)

	Argentina	ASU	London	New Zealand	Tanzania	Puerto Rico	Paraguay	North Phoenix	Nogales	Samoa	Iceland	All samples
People should eat what they feel like when they feel like it	F	F	F	F	F	F	F	F	F	F	F	F
If life is in balance, you have less risk of diabetes	T	T	T	T	T	T	T	T	T	T	T	T
Parents shouldn't worry too much about young children being overweight	F	F	F	F	T	F	F	F	50/50	F	F	F
STRUCTURAL FACTORS CREATE OBESITY												
Living in neighborhoods far away from super-markets contributes to people being fatter	F	F	F	F	F	F	F	F	F	F	F	F
You get really fat in the US because you can't walk anywhere	F	F	F	F	F	F	F	F	F	F	F	F
Being overweight is a sign of poverty	F	F	F	F	F	F	F	F	F	F	F	F
You get really fat in cities because you can't walk anywhere	F	F	F	F	T	F	F	F	T	F	F	F

People in cities tend to get fatter than people living in the countryside	T	F	T	T	T	T	T	T	F	F	T	F	T
Living close to parks or green spaces helps you stay fit and slim	F	T	F	T	T	T	F	F	T	F	F	F	F
America makes people fat	T	F	F	T	T	T	F	F	T	T	F	F	F
OVERWEIGHT/OBESITY IS BIOLOGICALLY "PROGRAMMED"													
Being overweight nowadays is normal	T	T	F	F	T	F	F	F	F	F	F	F	F
Some children are just born with a sweet-tooth	F	F	T	F	T	T	T	F	T	T	T	F	F
Overweight teens become overweight adults	T	T	T	T	F	T	T	T	T	T	T	T	T
If you are obese, it is because it is in your genes	F	F	F	F	T	F	F	F	F	F	F	F	F
Obesity and being overweight are genetic	F	F	F	F	F	50/50	F	F	F	F	F	F	F
Young children who are overweight will probably grow out of it	F	F	F	T	T	T	T	T	F	F	T	F	F

(continued)

TABLE D1

Results of a Cross-Cultural Survey and Consensus Analysis of Opinions on Obesity, 2009 *(continued)*

	Argentina	ASU	London	New Zealand	Tanzania	Puerto Rico	Paraguay	North Phoenix	Nogales	Samoa	Iceland	All samples
Some people are more predisposed genetically to obesity than others	T	T	T	T	T	T	T	T	T	T	T	T
Stress makes you gain weight	T	T	T	F	F	T	T	T	T	50/50	T	T
Obese people have different metabolisms	T	T	T	T	T	T	T	T	T	T	T	T
A baby cannot be overweight	F	F	F	F	F	F	T	F	F	F	F	F
Women get fatter after they have children	T	T	T	F	T	50/50	T	T	T	T	F	T
Men get fatter after they get married	T	T	T	F	T	F	T	T	T	T	F	T
It's easy to be slim if you want to be	F	F	F	F	F	F	T	F	T	T	F	F
OBESITY IS UNHEALTHY/ OBESITY IS A DISEASE												
Being overweight leads to diabetes	T	T	T	T	T	T	F	T	T	T	T	T

Being overweight will kill you	F	T	T	F	F	T	T	T	T	T	T	T
It is okay to gain a lot of weight while you are pregnant	F	F	F	F	F	F	F	F	F	F	F	F
Obesity is a very dangerous condition	T	T	T	T	T	T	T	T	T	T	T	T
Being a little overweight does not mean you are unhealthy	T	T	T	T	T	T	T	T	T	T	T	T
Medical insurance/the government shouldn't pay for obesity treatments	F	F	F	F	T	F	F	F	F	F	F	F
Obesity is a disease	T	T	T	50/50	F	T	T	T	T	T	T	T
Obesity is not a real medical condition	F	F	F	F	T	F	F	F	F	F	F	F
OBESITY/FAT IS BAD; SLIM IS GOOD												
If a child is chubby, a parent should be happy	F	F	F	F	T	F	F	F	F	F	F	F
For women, most things are in life are more important than being slim	F	T	T	T	T	T	T	T	T	T	T	T

(continued)

TABLE D1

Results of a Cross-Cultural Survey and Consensus Analysis of Opinions on Obesity, 2009 *(continued)*

	Argentina	ASU	London	New Zealand	Tanzania	Puerto Rico	Paraguay	North Phoenix	Nogales	Samoa	Iceland	All samples
Men find curvy women more attractive than slim ones	T	F	T	F	T	T	T	F	T	F	F	T
It is wrong to use elective surgery to make yourself slimmer	F	F	T	F	T	F	F	F	T	T	F	F
A skinny woman is not nearly as appealing as a wife	F	F	F	F	F	F	F	F	F	F	F	F
It is best to have an average sized body	T	T	T	T	T	T	T	T	T	T	T	T
Being skinny is a sign of poverty	F	F	F	F	F	F	F	F	F	F	F	F
Being fat is prestigious	F	F	F	F	F	F	F	F	F	F	F	F
People should be proud of their big bodies	F	F	F	F	F	F	F	F	F	T	F	F
Weight gain is a sign of contentment and happiness	F	F	F	F	F	F	F	F	F	F	F	F

Thin people are weak people	F	F	F	F	F	F	F	F	F	F	F	F	F
Obese people should be ashamed of their bodies	F	F	F	F	F	F	F	F	F	F	F	F	F
Chubby people deserve to be unhealthy	F	F	F	F	F	F	F	F	F	F	F	F	F
It's better to be chubby and happy	F	F	F	F	F	F	T	F	F	F	F	F	F
A beautiful woman has junk in the trunk or meat on her bones	F	F	F	T	F	F	F	F	F	F	T	F	F
The bigger the body, the greater the person	F	F	F	F	F	F	F	F	F	F	F	F	F
A big man is a powerful man	F	F	F	F	F	F	F	F	F	F	F	F	F
Chubby people tend to be happier than skinny people	F	F	F	F	F	F	F	F	F	F	F	F	F
A chubby child is a happy child	F	F	F	50/50	F	F	T	F	F	F	F	F	F
A person's weight means nothing	F	F	F	F	F	F	F	F	F	F	F	F	F
No one cares what people weigh	F	F	F	F	F	F	F	F	F	F	F	F	F

(continued)

TABLE D1

Results of a Cross-Cultural Survey and Consensus Analysis of Opinions on Obesity, 2009 *(continued)*

	Argentina	ASU	London	New Zealand	Tanzania	Puerto Rico	Paraguay	North Phoenix	Nogales	Samoa	Iceland	All samples
Being overweight makes for a less happy life	T	F	F	T	F	T	F	F	T	F	F	F
A big woman is a powerful woman	F	F	F	F	F	F	F	F	F	F	F	F
It's hard to make friends when you are significantly overweight	F	T	F	T	F	F	F	T	F	F	F	F
Fat people are lazy	F	F	F	F	F	F	T	F	T	T	F	F
Overweight people shouldn't be judged	T	T	T	T	T	T	T	T	T	T	T	T
Discrimination against people because they are obese is deplorable	T	T	T	T	T	T	T	T	T	T	T	T
You can never be too thin	F	F	F	F	F	F	F	F	F	F	F	F
If you are a little bit chubby, people will think less of you	F	F	F	F	F	F	F	F	50/50	F	F	F

Statement												Correct
You can tell a lot about someone by the size of their body	F	F	F	F	F	F	F	F	F	T	F	F
Being obese is harder for a woman than a man	F	T	F	T	F	T	F	T	T	T	F	F
A big woman is a beautiful woman	F	F	F	F	F	F	F	F	F	F	F	F
NOT CATEGORIZED												
Children shouldn't be on weight loss diets	F	T	T	T	T	T	T	T	T	T	T	T
Skipping meals is a good way to lose weight	F	F	F	F	F	F	F	F	F	F	F	F
Formula feeding can lead to babies gaining too much weight	F	F	F	F	F	F	F	F	F	F	F	F
Plastic surgery is a good idea when you want to get rid of excess weight	T	F	F	F	F	F	F	F	F	F	F	F

Note: The same questionnaire was used with each sample. The "culturally correct" answers for each country show differences in responses; the correct answer for the "global" model (all countries combined) appears in the column on the far right. For each statement, F = false, T = true; the designation usually means that the majority of people in the sample gave that answer, but in some cases (marked *) that people with high cultural knowledge tended to give that answer even if it was not a majority opinion.

border town of Nogales (mostly low-income Mexicans in the midst of the migration event); in relatively wealthy Scottsdale, Arizona; in urban Paraguay; London; Buenos Aires, Argentina; and with a sample of Arizona State University students. We included the undergraduate sample because the vast majority of the body image studies (including those done internationally) have been conducted with similar student populations. We then used Internet-based surveys combined with snowballing to gather samples from Puerto Rico, New Zealand, and Iceland. The final sample sizes and characteristics are given in table D2.

TABLE D2

Characteristics of Participants in a Cross-Cultural Study of Cultural Norms and Models Related to Obesity

	Sample Size (N)	% Female	Average Age	Average BMI	% Overweight (BMI > 25)
American Samoa	80	62.5	32.3	34.1	86.3
Argentina	40	50	32.4	23.4	28.2
ASU undergraduates	77	67.5	24.1	23.5	27.0
Iceland	86	66.3	32.4	25.8	49.4
London	66	40	34.5	23.9	40.6
Mexican border	46	34.8	45	28.3	75.6
New Zealand	44	70.5	51.9	23.7	27.3
Paraguay	105	69.2	37.2	25.9	53.8
Puerto Rico	52	63.5	37.3	26.9	51.9
Scottsdale, Arizona	44	61.4	37.2	23.6	27.3
Tanzania	40	57.5	46.9	25.3	48.5
Total	680	60	36.3	26.1	48.5

REFERENCES

Abdollahi, P., and T. Mann. 2001. Eating disorder symptoms and body image concerns in Iran: Comparisons between Iranian women in Iran and in America. *International Journal of Eating Disorders* 30:259–268.

Adams, G. R., M. Hicken, and M. Salehi. 1988. Socialization of the physical attractiveness stereotype: Parental expectations and verbal behaviors. *International Journal of Psychology* 23:137–149.

Akan, G. E., and C. M. Grilo. 1995. Sociocultural influences on eating attitudes and behaviors, body image, and psychological functioning: A comparison of African-American, Asian-American, and Caucasian college women. *International Journal of Eating Disorders* 18:181–187.

Albon, J. 1981. Stigmatized health conditions. *Social Science and Medicine* 15B: 5–9.

Allen, J. S., and S. M. Cheer. 1996. The non-thrifty genotype. *Current Anthropology* 37(5): 831–842.

Altabe, M. 1998. Ethnicity and body image: Quantitative and qualitative analysis. *International Journal of Eating Disorders* 23:153–159.

Anderson, N. B. 1999. Solving the puzzle of socioeconomic status and health: The need for integrated, multilevel, interdisciplinary research. *Annals of the New York Academy of Sciences* 896:302–312.

Anderson-Fye, E. P. 2004. A Coca-Cola shape: Cultural change, body image, and eating disorders in San Andrés, Belize. *Culture, Medicine, and Psychiatry* 28:561–595.

Angeles-Agdeppa, I., R. D. Lana, and C. V. C. Barba. 2003. A case study on dual forms of malnutrition among selected households in District 1, Tondo, Manila. *Asia Pacific Journal of Clinical Nutrition* 12:438–446.

Atlantis, E., and M. Baker. 2008. Obesity effects on depression: Systematic review of epidemiological studies. *International Journal of Obesity* 32(6): 881–891.

Auchincloss, A. H., and A. V. Diez Roux. 2008. A new tool for epidemiology? The usefulness of dynamic agent models in understanding place effects on health. *American Journal of Epidemiology* 168(1): 1–8.

Austin, J. L., and J. E. Smith. 2008. Thin ideal internalization in Mexican girls: A test of the sociocultural model of eating disorders. *International Journal of Eating Disorders* 41(5): 448–457.

Bacha, F., R. Saad, N. Gungor, J. Janosky, and S. A. Arslanian. 2003. Obesity, regional fat distribution, and syndrome X in obese black versus white adolescents: Race differential in diabetogenic and atherogenic risk factors. *Journal of Clinical Endocrinology and Metabolism* 88:2534–2540.

Baker, E. A., M. Schootman, E. Barnidge, and C. Kelly. 2006. The role of race and poverty in access to foods that enable individuals to adhere to dietary guidelines. *Preventing Chronic Disease* 3: A76.

Baker, P. T., J. M. Hanna, and T. S. Baker, eds. 1986. *The Changing Samoans: Behavior and Health in Transition.* New York: Oxford University Press.

Balsamo, A. 1996. *Technologies of the Gendered Body*. Durham, N.C.: Duke University Press.

Barak, Y., P. Sirpota, M. Tessler, A. Achiron, and Y. Lampl. 1994. Body esteem in Israeli university students. *Israel Journal of Psychiatry and Related Sciences* 31(4): 292–295.

Barker, D. 2001. *Fetal Origins of Cardiovascular and Lung Disease*. New York: Marcel Decker.

Bates, L. M., D. Acevedo-Garcia, M. Alegría, and N. Krieger. 2008. Immigration and generational trends in body mass index and obesity in the United States: Results of the National Latino and Asian American Survey, 2002–2003. *American Journal of Public Health* 98(1): 70–77.

Bateson, P., D. Barker, T. Clutton-Brock, D. Debal, B. D'Udine, R. A. Foley, P. Gluckman, K. Godfrey, T. Kirkwood, M. Mirazón Lahr, J. McNamara, N. B. Metcalfe, P. Monaghan, H. G. Spencer, and S. E. Sultan. 2004. Developmental plasticity and human health. *Nature* 430:419–421.

Bateson, P., and P. Martin. 1999. *Measuring Behavior*. Cambridge: Cambridge University Press.

Becker, A. E. 1995. *Body, Self, and Society: The View from Fiji*. Philadelphia: University of Pennsylvania Press.

———. 2004. Television, disordered eating, and young women in Fiji: Negotiating body image and identity during rapid social change. *Culture, Medicine, and Psychiatry* 28:533–559.

Becker, G. 1998. Coping with stigma: Lifelong adaptation of deaf people. In *Understanding and Applying Medical Anthropology*, ed. P. Brown, 311–316. London: Mayfield.

Becker, H. S. 1963. *Outsiders: Studies in the Sociology of Deviance*. New York: Free Press.

Berman, M. 2009. Africa—yes, Africa—has an obesity problem. *Newsweek*, http://www.newsweek.com/id/212556.

Berry, D., R. Sheehan, R. Heschel, K. Knafl, G. Melkus, and M. Grey. 2004. Family-based interventions for childhood obesity: A review. *Journal of Family Nursing* 10(4): 429–449.

Bilukha, O. O., and V. Utermohlen. 2002. Internalization of Western standards of appearance, body dissatisfaction, and dieting in urban educated Ukrainian females. *European Journal of Eating Disorders* 10:120–137.

Bindon, J. R., and P. T. Baker. 1985. Modernization, migration, and obesity among Samoan adults. *Annals of Human Biology* 12:67–76.

Björntorp, P. 2001. Do stress reactions cause abdominal obesity and comorbidities? *Obesity Review* 2(2): 73–86.

Blaine, B. 2008. Does depression cause obesity? A meta-analysis of longitudinal studies of depression and weight control. *Journal of Health Psychology* 13(8): 1190–1197.

Blair, S. N., and S. Brodney. 1999. Effects of physical inactivity and obesity on morbidity and mortality: Current evidence and research issues. *Medicine and Science in Sports and Exercise* 31: S646–S662.

Blane, D. 1995. Social determinants of health—Socioeconomic status, social class, and ethnicity. *American Journal of Public Health* 85(7): 903–904.

Bocquier, A., P. Verger, A. Basdevant, et al. 2005. Overweight and obesity: knowledge, attitudes, and practices of general practitioners in France. *Obesity Research* 13:787–795.

Bogin, N., and B. Beydoun. 2007. The relationship between sitting height ratio to body mass index in the United States, 1988–1994. *Human Ecology* 15:1–8.

Boone, C. 2008. Environmental justice as process and new avenues for research. *Environmental Justice* 1(3): 149–154.

Booth, K. M., M. M. Pinkston, and W.S.C. Poston. 2005. Obesity and the built environment. *Journal of the American Dietetic Association* 105:110–117.

Bordo, S. 1993. *Unbearable Weight: Feminism, Western Culture, and the Body*. Berkeley: University of California Press.

Bornstein, S., R. Schuppenies, A. Wong, and M. L. Licinio. 2006. Approaching the shared biology of obesity and depression: The stress axis as the locus of gene-environment interactions. *Molecular Psychiatry* 11:892–902.

Bouchard, C. 2007. The biological predisposition to obesity: Beyond the thrifty genotype scenario. *International Journal of Obesity* 31:1337–1339.

Bray, G. A. 1987. Obesity: A disease of nutrient or energy balance? *Nutrition Reviews* 45: 33–43.

Bray, G. A., S. J. Nielsen, and B. M. Popkin. 2004. Consumption of high-fructose corn syrup in beverages may play a role in the epidemic of obesity. *American Journal of Clinical Nutrition* 79(4): 537–543.

Bray, G. A., and B. M. Popkin. 1998. Dietary fat intake does affect obesity! *American Journal of Clinical Nutrition* 68:1157–1173.

Brewis, A. 2003. Biocultural aspects of obesity in young Mexican schoolchildren. *American Journal of Human Biology* 15(3): 446–460.

Brewis, A., and M. Gartin. 2006. Biocultural construction of obesogenic ecologies of childhood: Parent-feeding versus child-eating strategies. *American Journal of Human Biology* 18(2): 203–213.

Brewis, A., G. Irwin, and J. S. Allen. 1995. Patterns of colonisation and the "thrifty" genotype in Pacific prehistory. *Asia Pacific Journal of Clinical Nutrition* 4: 361–365.

Brewis, A., and S. Lee 2010. Children's work, earnings, and nutrition in urban Mexican shantytowns. *American Journal of Human Biology* 22(1): 60–68.

Brewis, A., and S. T. McGarvey. 2000. Body image, body size and Samoan ecological and individual modernization. *Ecology of Food and Nutrition* 39:105–120.

Brewis, A., S. T. McGarvey, J. Jones, and B. A. Swinburn. 1998. Perceptions of body size in Pacific Islanders. *International Journal of Obesity* 22(2): 185–189.

Brewis, A., and K. L. Schmidt. 2003. Gender variation in the identification of Mexican children's psychiatric symptoms. *Medical Anthropology Quarterly* 17(3): 376–393.

Brink, P. J. 1989. The fattening room among the Annang of Nigeria. *Medical Anthropology* 12:131–143.

Brochu, M., A. Tchernof, I. J. Dionne, C. K. Sites, G. H. Eltabbakh, E.A.H. Sims, and E. T. Poehlman. 2001. What are the physical characteristics associated with a normal metabolic profile despite a high level of obesity in postmenopausal women? *Journal of Clinical Endocrinology and Metabolism* 86:1020–1025.

Brown, P. J., and M. Konner. 1987. An anthropological perspective of obesity. *Annals of the New York Academy of Science* 499:29–46.

Brown, P. J., and S. V. Krick. 2001. Culture and ethnicity in the etiology of obesity: Diet, television, and the illusion of personal choice. In *Obesity, Physical Growth, and Development*, ed. F. E. Johnston and G. Foster, 111–157. London: Smith-Gordo.

Brown, P. J., and J. Sweeney. 2009. The anthropology of overweight, obesity, and the body. *AnthroNotes* 30(1): 6–12.

Bulik, C. M., L. Reba, A. M. Siega-Riz, and T. Reichborn-Kjennerud. 2005. Anorexia nervosa: Definition, epidemiology and cycle of risk. *International Journal of Eating Disorders* 37: S2–S9.

Bulik, C. M., T. D. Wade, A. C. Heath, N. G. Martin, A. J. Stunkard, and L. J. Eaves. 2001. Relating body mass index to figural stimuli: Population-based normative data for Caucasians. *International Journal of Obesity Related Metabolic Disorders* 25(10): 1517–1524.

Burt, R. S. 1984. Network items and the general social survey. *Social Networks* 6:293–340.

Buss, D. 1989. Sex differences in human mate preferences: Evolutionary hypotheses tested in 37 cultures. *Behavior, Brain, and Science* 12:1–49.

Caballero, B. 2005. A nutrition paradox: Underweight and obesity in developing countries. *New England Journal of Medicine* 352:1514–1516.

Cachelin, F. M., R. M. Rebeck, G. H. Chung, and E. Pelayo. 2002. Does ethnicity influence body-size preference? A comparison of body image and body size. *Obesity* 10(3): 158–166.

Caldwell, M. B., K. D. Brownell, and D. E. Wilfley. 1997. Relationship of weight, body dissatisfaction, and self-esteem in African American and white female dieters. *International Journal of Eating Disorders* 22:127–130.

Calle, E. E., M. J. Thun, J. M. Petrelli, C. Rodriguez, and C. W. Heath. 1999. Body-mass index and mortality in a prospective cohort of U.S. Adults. *New England Journal of Medicine* 341:1097–1105.

Campbell, K., H. Engel, A. Timperio, C. Cooper, and D. Crawford. 2000. Obesity management: Australian general practitioners' attitudes and practices. *Obesity Research* 8:459–466.

Campbell, K., E. Waters, S. O'Meara, and C. Summerbell. 2001. Interventions for preventing obesity in childhood: A systematic review. *Obesity Reviews* 2(3): 149–157.

Campos, P. 2004. *The Obesity Myth: Why America's Obsession with Weight Is Hazardous to Your Health.* New York: Penguin.

Campos, P., A. Saguy, P. Ernsberger, E. Oliver, and G. Gaesser. 2006. The epidemiology of overweight and obesity: Public health crisis or moral panic? *International Journal of Epidemiology* 35(1): 55–60.

Caprio, S., S. R. Daniels, A. Drewnowski, F. R. Kaufman, L. A. Palinkas, A. L. Rosenbloom, and J. B. Schwimmer. 2008. Influence of race, ethnicity, and culture on childhood obesity: Implications for prevention and treatment. A consensus statement of Shaping America's Health and the Obesity Society. *Diabetes Care* 31(11): 2211–2221.

Caputi, J. 1983. One size does not fit all: Being beautiful, thin, and female in America. In *The Popular Culture Reader*, 3rd ed., ed. J. Nachbar and C. Geist, 186–204. Bowling Green, Ohio: Popular Press.

Carr, D., and M. A. Friedman. 2005. Is obesity stigmatizing? Body weight, perceived discrimination, and psychological well-being in the United States. *Journal of Health and Social Behavior* 46:244–259.

Carryer, J. 1997. Embodied largeness: A feminist exploration. In *Bodily Boundaries, Sexualized Genders, Medical Discourses*, ed. M. De Ras and V. Grace. Wellington, New Zealand: Dunmore Press.

———. 2001. Embodied largeness: A significant women's health issue. *Nursing Inquiry* 8:90–97.

CDC [Centers for Disease Control and Prevention]. 2008a. "NCHS data on racial and ethnic disparities." National Center for Health Statistics information sheet. http://www.cdc.gov/nchs/data/infosheets/infosheet_race_ethnicity.htm.

———. 2008b. Behavioral Risk Factor Surveillance System. "U.S. obesity trends." http://www.cdc.gov/obesity/data/trends.html#State.

Chambliss, H. O., C. E. Finley, and S. N. Blair. 2004. Attitudes toward obese individuals among exercise science students. *Medicine and Science in Sports and Exercise* 36(3): 468–474.

Chang, V., and N. Christakis. 2002. Medical modeling of obesity: A transition from action to experience in a 20th century American medical textbook. *Sociology of Health and Illness* 24:151–177.

Chin-Hong, P. V., and S. T. McGarvey. 1996. Lifestyle incongruity and adult blood pressure in Western Samoa. *Psychosomatic Medicine* 58(2): 131–137.

Christakis, N. A., and J. H. Fowler. 2007. The spread of obesity in a large social network over 32 years. *New England Journal of Medicine* 357(4): 370–379.

Cohn, L. D., and N. E. Adler. 1992. Female and male perceptions of ideal body shapes. *Psychology of Women Quarterly* 16:69–79.

Cohn, L. D., N. E. Adler, C. E. Irwin Jr., S. G. Millstein, S. M. Kegeles, and G. Stone. 1987. Body-figure preferences in male and female adolescents. *Journal of Abnormal Psychology* 96(3): 276–279.

Cole, T. J., M. C. Bellizzi, K. M. Flegal, and W. H. Dietz. 2000. Establishing a standard definition for child overweight and obesity worldwide: International survey. *British Medical Journal* 320:1240–1243.

Collins, P. H. 2000. Gender, black feminism, and black political economy. *Annals of the American Academy of Political and Social Science* 568:41–53.

Cordain, L., S. Boyd Eaton, A. Sebastian, N. Mann, S. Lindeberg, B. A. Watkins, J. H. O'Keefe, and J. B. Miller. 2005. Origins and evolution of the western diet: Health implications for the 21st century. *American Journal of Clinical Nutrition* 81:341–354.

Cordell, G., and C. R. Ronai. 1999. Identity management among overweight women: Narrative resistance to stigma. In *Interpreting Weight: The Social Management of Fatness and Thinness*, ed. J. Sobal and D. Maurer, 29–48. New York: Aldine de Gruyter.

Cornelissen, P. L., M. J. Toveé, and M. Bateson. 2009. Patterns of subcutaneous fat deposition and the relationship between body mass index and waist-to-hip ratio: Implications for models of physical attractiveness. *Journal of Theoretical Biology* 256(3): 343–350.

Couzin, J. 2005. Public health: A heavyweight battle over CDC's obesity forecasts. *Science* 308(5723): 770–771.

Coyne, T. 2000. *Obesity in the Pacific: Too Big to Ignore.* Secretariat of the Pacific Community, Noumea.

Craig, P. L., V. Halavatau, E. Comino, and I. Caterson. 1999. Perception of body size in the Tongan community: Differences from and similarities to an Australian sample. *International Journal of Obesity* 23:1288–1294.

———. 2001. Differences in body composition between Tongans and Australians: Time to rethink the healthy weight ranges? *International Journal of Obesity* 25: 1806–1814.

Crandall, C. S. 1994. Prejudice against fat people: Ideology and self-interest. *Journal of Personality and Social Psychology* 66:882–894.

———. 1995. Do parents discriminate against their heavyweight daughters? *Personality and Social Psychology Bulletin* 21:724–735.

Crandall, C. S., S. D'Anello, N. Sakalli, E. Lazarus, G. W. Nejtardt, and N. T. Feather. 2001. An attribution-value model of prejudice: Anti-fat attitudes in six nations. *Personality and Social Psychology Bulletin* 27:30–37.

Crandall, C. S., and R. Martinez. 1996. Culture, ideology, and anti-fat attitudes. *Personality and Social Psychology Bulletin* 22:1165–1176.

Crespo, C. E., E. Smit, O. Carter-Pokras, and R. Andersen. 2001. Acculturation and leisure-time physical inactivity in Mexican American adults: Results from NHANES III, 1988–1994. *American Journal of Public Health* 91(8): 1254–1257.

Critser, G. 2003. *Fat Land: How Americans Became the Fattest People in the World.* Boston and New York: Houghton Mifflin.

Crooks, D. L. 1998. Poverty and nutrition in eastern Kentucky: The political-economy of childhood growth. In *Building a New Biocultural Synthesis: Political-Economic Perspectives on Human Biology*, ed. A. H. Goodman and T. L. Leatherman, 339–355. Ann Arbor: University of Michigan Press.

———. 2003. Trading nutrition for education: Nutritional status and the sale of snack foods in an eastern Kentucky school. *Medical Anthropology Quarterly* 17:182–199.

Crooks, D. L., L. Cliggett, and S. M. Cole. 2007. Child growth as a measure of livelihood security: The case of the Gwembe Tonga. *American Journal of Human Biology* 19(5): 669–675.

Csordas, T. J. 1990. Embodiment as a paradigm for anthropology. *Ethos* 18:5–47.

Cummins, S., and S. Macintyre. 2002. 'Food deserts'—evidence and assumption in policy making. *British Medical Journal* 325:436–438.

———. 2006. Food environments and obesity—neighborhoods or nation? *International Journal of Epidemiology* 35:100–104.

Cummins, S., M. Petticrew, C. Higgins, A. Findlay, and L. Sparks. 2005. Large-scale food retailing as a health intervention: Quasi-experimental evaluation of a natural experiment. *Journal of Epidemiology and Community Health* 59:1035–1040.

Cutler, D. M., E. L. Glaeser, and J. M. Shapiro. 2003. Why have Americans become more obese? *Journal of Economic Perspectives* 17:93–118.

Cutts, B., K. Darby, C. Boone, and A. Brewis. 2009. City structure, obesity, and environmental justice: An integrated analysis of physical and social barriers to walkable streets and park access. *Social Science and Medicine* 69(9): 1314–1322.

Dabelea, D., D. J. Pettitt, R. L. Hanson, G. Imperatore, P. H. Bennett, and W. C. Knowler. 1999. Birth weight, type 2 diabetes, and insulin resistance in Pima Indian children and young adults. *Diabetes Care* 22:944–950.

Danadian, K., V. Lewy, J. J. Janosky, and S. Arslanian. 2001. Lipolysis in African-American children: Is it a metabolic risk factor predisposing to obesity? *Journal of Clinical Endocrinology and Metabolism* 86(7): 3022–3026.

de Garine, I., and N. J. Pollock. 1995. *Social Aspects of Obesity*. Amsterdam: Gordon and Breach.

Degher, D., and G. Hughes. 1999. The adoption and management of a "fat" identity. In *Interpreting Weight: The Social Management of Fatness and Thinness*, ed. J. Sobal and D. Maurer, 11–27. New York: Aldine de Gruyter.

DeJong, W. 1993. Obesity as a characterological stigma: The issue of responsibility and judgments of task performance. *Psychological Reports* 73:963–970.

Demarest, J., and R. Allen. 2000. Body image: Gender, ethnic, and age differences. *Journal of Social Psychology* 140:465–472.

DeMattia, L., and S. L. Denney. 2008. Childhood obesity prevention: Successful community-based efforts. *Annals of the American Academy of Political and Social Science* 615:83–99.

Desmond, S., J. Price, C. Hallinan, and D. Smith. 1989. Black and white adolescents' perceptions of their weight. *Journal of School Health* 59:353–358.

Deurenberg, P., M. Yap, and W. A. van Staveren. 1998. Body mass index and percent body fat: A meta analysis among different ethnic groups. *International Journal of Obesity and Related Metabolic Disorders* 22(12): 1164–1171.

Deurenberg-Yap, M. 2000. Body composition and diet of Chinese, Malays and Indians in Singapore. PhD diss., Wageningen University.

de Vries, J. 2007. The obesity epidemic: Medical and ethical considerations. *Science and Engineering Ethics* 13(1): 55–67.

Dierk, J. M., M. Conradt , E. Rauh, P. Schlumberger, J. Hebebrand, and W. Rief. 2006. What determines well-being in obesity? Associations with BMI, social skills, and social support. *Journal of Psychosomatic Research* 60(3): 219–227.

Dietz, W. H. 1997. Periods of risk in childhood for the development of adult obesity—what do we need to learn? *Journal of Nutrition* 127(9): S1884–S1886.

———. 1998. Health consequences of obesity in youth: Childhood predictors of adult disease. *Pediatrics* 101(3): 518–525.

Dixson, B. J., A. F. Dixson, B. Li, and M. J. Anderson. 2007. Studies of human physique and sexual attractiveness: Sexual preferences of men and women in China. *American Journal of Human Biology* 19(1): 88–95.

Doak, C. M., L. Adair, M. Bentley, C. Monteiro, and B. M. Popkin. 2002 The nutrition transition and the underweight/overweight household: A seven-country comparison. *FASEB Journal* 16: A615–A616.

———. 2005. The dual burden household and the nutrition transition paradox. *International Journal of Obesity* 29:129–136.

Doak, C., L. Adair, M. Bentley, F. Y. Zhai, and B. Popkin. 2002. The underweight/overweight household: an exploration of household sociodemographic and dietary factors in China. *Public Health Nutrition* 5:215–221.

Doak, C. M., L. Adair, C. Monteiro, and B. M. Popkin. 2000. Overweight and underweight coexist within households in Brazil, China, and Russia. *Journal of Nutrition* 130:2965–2971.

Douglas, M. 1970. *Natural Symbols: Explorations in Cosmology.* New York: Routledge.

Doyle, S., A. Kelly-Schwartz, and M. Schlossberg. 2006. Active community environments and health: The relationship of walkable and safe communities to individual health. *Journal of the American Planning Association* 72(1): 19–31.

Dressler, W. W. 1995. Modeling biocultural interactions: Examples from studies of stress and cardiovascular disease. *American Journal of Physical Anthropology* 38(S21): 27–56.

———. 1999. Modernization, stress and blood pressure: New directions in research. *Human Biology* 71:583–605.

———. 2004. Culture and the risk of disease. *British Medical Bulletin* 69:21–31.

Dressler, W. W., K. S. Oths, and C. C. Gravlee. 2005. Race and ethnicity in public health research: Models to explain health disparities. *Annual Review of Anthropology* 34(1): 231–252.

Dressler, W. W., K. Oths, R. Ribeiro, M. Balieiro, and J. Dos Santos. 2008. Cultural consonance and adult body composition in urban Brazil. *American Journal of Human Biology* 20:15–22.

Du, S., T. A. Mroz, F. Zhai, and B. M. Popkin. 2004. Rapid income growth adversely affects diet quality in China—particularly for the poor! *Social Science and Medicine* 59(7): 1505–1515.

Dubois, L., A. Farmer, M. Girard, and M. Porcherie. 2006. Family food insufficiency is related to overweight among preschoolers. *Social Science and Medicine* 63(6): 1503–1516.

Dufour, D. L., and B. A. Piperata. 2008. Energy expenditure among farmers in developing countries: What do we know? *American Journal of Human Biology* 20:249–258.

Eaton, S. B., and M. Konner. 1985. Paleolithic nutrition: A consideration of its nature and current implications. *New England Journal of Medicine* 312(5): 283–289.

Eaton, S. B., M. Konner, and M. Shostak. 1988. Stone-agers in the fast lane: Chronic degenerative diseases in evolutionary perspective. *American Journal of Medicine* 84:739–749.

Edwards, P., and I. Roberts. 2009. Population adiposity and climate change. *International Journal of Epidemiology* 38(4): 1137–1140.

Egger, G., and B. Swinburn. 1997. An 'ecological' approach to the obesity pandemic. *British Medical Journal* 315:477–480.

Eisenberg, M. E., D. Neumark-Sztainer, and M. Story. 2003. Associations of weight-based teasing and emotional well-being among adolescents. *Archives of Pediatrics and Adolescent Medicine* 157:733–738.

Ellison, P. 2003. *On Fertile Ground: A Natural History of Human Reproduction.* Cambridge, Mass.: Harvard University Press.

Emmons, K. M. 2000. Health behaviours in a social context. In *Social Epidemiology*, ed. L. F. Berkman and I. Kawachi, 242–266. Oxford: Oxford University Press.

Eveleth, P. B., and J. M. Tanner. 1976. *Worldwide Variation in Human Growth.* Cambridge: Cambridge University Press.

Ewing, R., T. Schmid, R. Killingsworth, A. Zlot, and S. Raudenbush. 2003. Relationship between urban sprawl and physical activity, obesity, and morbidity. *American Journal of Health Promotion* 18(1): 47–57.

Ezzati, M., S. Vander Hoorn, C. M. M. Lawes, R. Leach, W.P.T. James, A. D. Lopez, A. Rodgers, and C.J.L. Murray. 2005. Rethinking the diseases of affluence paradigm: Global patterns of nutrition risks in relation to economic development. *PLoS Medicine* 2(5): e133.

Fallon, A., and P. Rozin. 1985. Sex differences in perceptions of desirable body shape. *Journal of Personality and Social Psychology* 94:102–105.

Fantuzzi, G. 2009. Tuberculosis and the inflammatory processes of obesity in human evolution. *Journal of the American Medical Association* 302(916): 1754–1755.

Farmer, P. 1999. *Infections and Inequalities: The Modern Plagues.* Berkeley: University of California Press.

———. 2005. *Pathologies of Power.* Berkeley: University of California Press.

Fingeret, M. C., D. H. Gleaves, and C. A. Pearson. 2004. On the methodology of body image assessment: The use of figural rating scales to evaluate body dissatisfaction and the ideal body standards of women. *Body Image* 1:207–212.

Finkelstein, E. A., I. Fiebelkorn, and G. Wang. 2003. National medical spending attributable to overweight and obesity: How much, and who's paying. *Health Affairs* 3(1): 219–226.

Flegal, K. M., C. L. Ogden, and M. Carroll. 2004. Prevalence and trends in overweight in Mexican-American adults and children. *Nutrition Reviews* 62: S144–S148.

Florencio, T., H. Ferreira, A.P.T. de Franca, J. C. Cavalcante, and A. L. Sawaya. 2001. Obesity and undernutrition in a very-low-income population in the city of Maceio, northeastern Brazil. *British Journal of Nutrition* 86:277–283.

Foerster, S. B., and M. Hudes. 1989. *California Dietary Practices Survey: Focus on Fruits and Vegetables—Final Report.* Sacramento, Calif.: Nutrition and Cancer Prevention Program, California Department of Health Services.

Fogelman, Y., S. Vinker, and J. Lachter. 2002. Managing obesity: A survey of attitudes and practices among Israeli primary care physicians. *International Journal of Obesity* 26:1393–1397.

Forbes, G. B., L. Adams-Curtis, R. L. Jobe, K. B. White, J. Revak, I. Zivcic-Becirevic, and A. Pokrajac-Bulian. 2005. Body dissatisfaction in college women and their mothers: Cohort effects, developmental effects, and the influences of body size, sexism, and the thin body ideal. *Sex Roles* 53(3–4): 281–298.

Ford, E. S., W. H. Giles, and W. H. Dietz. 2002. Prevalence of the metabolic syndrome among U.S. adults: Findings from the Third National Health and Nutrition Examination Survey. *Journal of the American Medical Association* 287:356–359.

Ford, K. A., B. M. Dolan, and C. Evans. 1990. Cultural factors in the eating disorders: A study of body shape preferences of Arab students. *Journal of Psychosomatic Research* 34(5): 501–507.

Ford, P. B., and D. A. Dzewaltowski. 2008. Disparities in obesity prevalence due to variation in the retail food environment: Three testable hypotheses. *Nutrition Reviews* 66:216–228.

Foster, G. D., T. A. Wadden, A. P. Makris, D. Davidson, R. S. Sanderson, D. B. Allison, and A. Kessler. 2003. Primary care physicians' attitudes about obesity and its treatment. *Obesity Research* 11(10): 1168–1177.

Foucault, M. 1972. *The Archaeology of Knowledge.* Translated by A. M. Sheridan Smith. London: Tavistock.

Freedman, D. S., L. K. Khan, M. K. Serdula, C. L. Ogden, and W. H. Dietz. 2006. Racial and ethnic differences in secular trends for childhood BMI, weight, and height. *Obesity* 14:301–308.

French, S. A., M. Story, and R. W. Jeffery. 2001. Environmental influences on eating and physical activity. *Annual Review of Public Health* 22(1): 309–335.

Frias-Armenta, M., and L. McCloskey. 1998. Determinants of harsh parenting in Mexico. *Behavioral Science* 26(2): 129–139.

Friedman, J. M. 2003. A war of obesity, not the obese. *Science* 299(5608): 856–858.

Frisancho, A. R. 1993. *Human Adaptation and Accommodation.* Ann Arbor: University of Michigan Press.

———. 2003. Reduced rate of fat oxidation: A metabolic pathway to obesity in the developing nations. *American Journal of Human Biology* 15:522–532.

Frisch, R. E. 1990. Body fat, menarche, fitness, and fertility. In *Adipose Tissue and Reproduction*, ed. R. E. Frisch, 1–26. Basel, Switzerland: Karger.

Furnham, A., and N. Alibhai. 1983. Cross cultural differences in the perception of female body shape. *Psychological Medicine* 13:829–837.

Furnham, A., N. Badmin, and I. Sneade. 2002. Body image dissatisfaction: Gender differences in eating attitudes, self-esteem, and reasons for exercise. *Journal of Psychology* 36(6): 581–596.

Furnham, A., and P. Baguma. 1994. Cross-cultural differences in the evaluation of male and female body shapes. *International Journal of Eating Disorders* 15:81–89.

Furnham, A., C. Hester, and C. Weir. 1990. Sex differences in the preferences for specific female body shapes. *Sex Roles* 22(11–12): 679–797.

Furnham, A., and S. Radley. 1989. Sex differences in the perception of male and female body shapes. *Personality and Individual Differences* 10:653–662.

Furnham, A., T. Tan, and C. McManus. 1997. Waist-to-hip ratio and preferences for body shape: A replication and extension. *Personal and Individual Differences* 22: 539–549.

Gaesser, G. A. 2003. Weight, weight loss, and health: A closer look at the evidence. *Healthy Weight Journal* 17(1): 8–11.

Galanis, D., P. Chin-Hong, S. McGarvey, E. Messer, and D. Parkinson. 1995. Dietary changes associated with post-cyclone food aid in Western Samoa. *Ecology of Food and Nutrition* 34:137–145.

Gallagher, M. 2006. *Examining the Impact of Food Deserts on Public Health in Chicago*. Chicago: Mari Gallagher Research and Consulting Group.

Gampel, B. 1962. The "Hilltops" Community. In *Practice of Social Medicine*, ed. S. Kark and G. Steuart, 292–308. Edinburgh and London: E. and S. Livingston.

Gard, M., and J. Wright. 2005. *The Obesity Epidemic: Science, Morality and Ideology*. London: Routledge.

Garrett, J., and M. T. Ruel. 2005. The coexistence of child undernutrition and maternal overweight: Prevalence, hypotheses, and programme and policy implications. *Maternal and Child Nutrition* 1(3): 185–196.

Garrow, J. S., and J. Webster. 1985. Quetelet's index (W/H^2) as a measure of fatness. *International Journal of Obesity* 9:147–153.

Gelber, R. P., J. M. Gaziano, E. J. Orav, J. E. Manson, J. E. Buring, and T. Kurth. 2008. Measures of obesity and cardiovascular risk among men and women. *Journal of the American College of Cardiology* 52(8): 605–615.

Germov, J., and L. Williams. 1999. Dieting women: Self-surveillance and the body panopticon. In *Weighty Issues: Fatness and Thinness as Social Problems*, ed. J. Sobal and D. Maurer, 117–132. New York: Aldine de Gruyter.

Giammattei, J., G. Blix, H. Hopp, A. Marshak, O. Wollitzer, and D. J. Pettitt. 2003. Television watching and soft drink consumption: Associations with obesity in 11- to 13-year-old schoolchildren. *Archives of Pediatrics and Adolescent Medicine* 157:882–886.

Gibbs, W. W. 2005. Obesity: An overblown epidemic? *Scientific American* 292(6): 70–76.

Giles-Corti, B., M. H. Broomhall, M. Knuiman, C. Collins, K. Douglas, A. Lange, and R. Donovan. 2005. Increasing walking—how important is distance to, attractiveness, and size of public open space? *American Journal of Preventive Medicine* 28(2): 169–176.

Giles-Corti, B., and R. J. Donovan 2002. The relative influence of individual, social, and physical environment determinants of physical activity. *Social Science and Medicine* 54:1793–1812.

Giles-Corti, B., S. Macintyre, J. P. Clarkson, T. Pikora, and R. J. Donovan. 2003. Environmental and lifestyle factors associated with overweight and obesity in Perth, Australia. *American Journal of Health Promotion* 18:93–102.

Gittelsohn, J., S. B. Harris, A. L. Thorne-Lyman, A. J. Hanley, A. Barnie, and B. Zinman. 1996. Body image concepts differ by age and sex in an Ojibway-Cree community in Canada. *Journal of Nutrition* 126(12): 2990–3000.

Gluckman, P., and M. Hanson. 2005. *The Fetal Matrix: Evolution, Development, and Disease.* Cambridge: Cambridge University Press.

Goel, M. S., E. P. McCarthy, R. S. Phillips, and C. C. Wee. 2004. Obesity among U.S. immigrant subgroups by duration of residence. *Journal of the American Medical Association* 292(23): 2860–67.

Goffman, E. 1963. *Stigma: Notes on the Management of Spoiled Identity.* New York: Prentice-Hall.

Goldblatt, P., M. Moore, and A. Stunkard. 1965. Social factors in obesity. *Journal of the American Medical Association* 192(12): 1039–1044.

Good, B. 1994. *Medicine, Rationality, and Experience: An Anthropological Perspective.* Cambridge: Cambridge University Press.

Goran, M., R. N. Bergman, M. L. Cruz, and R. Watanabe. 2002. Insulin resistance and associated compensatory responses in African-American and Hispanic children. *Diabetes Care* 25(12): 2184–2190.

Gordon-Larsen, P., K. M. Harris, D. S. Ward, and B. M. Popkin. 2003. Acculturation and overweight-related behaviors among Hispanic immigrants to the U.S.: The National Longitudinal Study of Adolescent Health. *Social Science and Medicine* 57:2023–2034.

Gordon-Larsen, P., M. Nelson, P. Page, and B. Popkin. 2006. Inequality in the built environment underlies key health disparities in physical activity and obesity. *Pediatrics* 117(2): 417–424.

Gould, P. 1994. Polynesian body image and body size: Transformations and implications. Master's thesis, University of Auckland.

Gravlee, C. C. 2009. How race becomes biology: Embodiment of social inequality. *American Journal of Physical Anthropology* 139(1): 47–57.

Gravlee, C. C., W. W. Dressler, and H. R. Bernard. 2005. Skin color, social classification, and blood pressure in Puerto Rico. *American Journal of Public Health* 95(12): 2191–2197.

Greenberg, D., and D. LaPorte. 1996. Racial differences in body type preferences of men for women. *International Journal of Eating Disorders* 19:275–278.

Gremillion, H. 2005. The cultural politics of body size. *Annual Reviews in Anthropology* 34:13–32.

Grineski, S., B. Bolin, and C. G. Boone. 2007. Criteria air pollution and marginalized populations: Environmental inequity in metropolitan Phoenix, Arizona, USA. *Social Science Quarterly* 88(2): 535–554.

Grogan, S., and H. Richards. 2002. Body image: Focus groups with boys and men. *Men and Masculinities* 4:219–233.

Grün, F., and B. Blumberg. 2006. Environmental obesogens: Organotins and endocrine disruption via nuclear receptor signaling. *Endocrinology* 147(6): s50–s55.

———. 2009. Minireview: The case for obesogens. *Molecular Endocrinology* 23(8): 1127–1134.

Gu, D., J. He, X. Duan, K. Reynolds, X. Wu, J. Chen, G. Huang, C. S. Chen, and P. K. Whelton. 2006. Body weight and mortality among men and women in China. *Journal of the American Medical Association* 295(7): 776–783.

Hadley, C., A. Brewis, and I. Pike. 2010. Does less autonomy erode women's health? Yes. No. Maybe. *American Journal of Human Biology* 22(1): 103–110.

Hadley, C., and C. Patil. 2006. Food insecurity in rural Tanzania is associated with maternal anxiety and depression. *American Journal of Human Biology* 18(3): 359–368.

Haile, B. J., and A. E. Johnson. 1989. Teaching and learning about black women: The anatomy of a course. *Scholarly Journal of Black Women* 6:69–73.

Hales, C. N., and D. J. Barker. 1992. Type 2 (non-insulin-dependent) diabetes mellitus: The thrifty phenotype hypothesis. *Diabetologia* 35:595–601.

Hanna, J. M., D. L. Pelletier, and V. J. Brown. 1986. The diet and nutrition of contemporary Samoans. In *The Changing Samoans: Behavior and Health in Transition*, ed. P. T. Baker, J. M. Hanna, and T. S. Baker, 275–296. New York: Oxford University Press.

Hannon, B. M., and T. G. Lohman. 1978. The energy cost of overweight in the United States. *American Journal of Public Health* 68(8): 765–767.

Harkness, S., and C. M. Super. 1994. The "developmental niche": A theoretical framework for analyzing the household production of health. *Social Science and Medicine* 38(2): 217–226.

Hartley, C. 2001. Letting ourselves go: Making room for the fat body in feminist scholarship. In *Bodies Out of Bounds: Fatness and Transgression*, ed. J. E. Braziel and K. LeBesco, 60–73. Berkeley: University of California Press.

Harvey, E. L., and A. J. Hill. 2001. Health professionals' views of overweight people and smokers. *International Journal of Obesity and Related Metabolic Disorders* 25:1253–1261.

Henriques, G. R., and L. G. Calhoun. 1999. Gender and ethnic differences in the relationship between body esteem and self-esteem. *Journal of Psychology* 133:357–368.

Herbozo, S., S. Tantleff-Dunn, J. Gokee-Larose, and J. K. Thompson. 2004. Beauty and thinness messages in children's media: A content analysis. *Eating Disorders* 12:21–34.

Hill, J. O., H. R. Wyatt, G. W. Reed, and J. C. Peters. 2003. Obesity and the environment: Where do we go from here? *Science* 299:853–855.

Hill, K., K. Hawkes, M. Hurtado, and H. Kaplan. 1984. Seasonal variance in the diet of Ache hunter-gatherers in Eastern Paraguay. *Human Ecology* 12(2): 101–135.

Hill, M. 1997. The diabetes epidemic in Indian country. *Winds of Change, American Indian Science and Engineering Quarterly* (summer): 26–31.

Hillsdon, M., N. Cavill, K. Nanchahal, A. Diamond, and I. R. White. 2001. National level promotion of physical activity: Results from England's ACTIVE for LIFE campaign. *Journal of Epidemiology and Community Health* 55:755–761.

Himmelgreen, D. A., R. Perez-Escamilla, D. Martinez, A. Bretnall, B. Eells, and Y. Peng. 2004. The longer you stay, the bigger you get: Length of time and language use in the U.S. are associated with obesity in Puerto Rican women. *American Journal of Physical Anthropology* 125:90–96.

Hoffman, D. J., A. L. Sawaya, W. A. Coward, A. Wright, P. A. Martins, C. De Nascimento, K. L. Tucker, and S. B. Roberts. 2000. Energy expenditure of stunted and non-stunted boys and girls living in the shantytowns of Sao Paulo, Brazil. *American Journal of Clinical Nutrition* 72:1025–1031.

Honeycutt, K. 1999. Fat world/thin world: "Fat busters," "equivocators," "fat boosters," and the social construction of obesity. In *Interpreting Weight: The Social Management of Fatness and Thinness*, ed. J. Sobal and D. Maurer, 165–182. New York: Aldine de Gruyter.

Horowitz, C. R., K. Colson, P. Hebert, and K. Lancaster. 2004. Barriers to buying healthy foods for people with diabetes: Evidence of environmental disparities. *American Journal of Public Health* 94:1549–1554.

Houghton, P. 1991. The early human biology of the Pacific: Some considerations. *Journal of the Polynesian Society* 100(2): 167–196.

Howard, A. 1986. Questions and answers: Samoans talk about happiness, distress, and other life experiences. In *The Changing Samoans: Behavior and Health in Transition*, ed. P. Baker, J. Hanna, and T. Baker, 174–202. New York: Oxford University Press.

Hruschka, D. J., L. M. Sibley, N. Kalim, and J. K. Edmonds. 2008. When there is more than one answer key: Cultural theories of postpartum hemorrhage in Matlab, Bangladesh. *Field Methods* 20(4): 315–337.

Hsieh, S. D., and T. Muto. 2006. Metabolic syndrome in Japanese men and women with special reference to the anthropometric criteria for the assessment of obesity: Proposal to use the waist-to-height ratio. *American Journal of Preventive Medicine* 42:135–139.

Hu, F. B, W. C Willett, T. Li, M. J. Stampfer, G. A. Colditz, and J. E. Manson. 2004. Adiposity as compared with physical activity in predicting mortality among women. *New England Journal of Medicine* 351(6): 2694–2703.

Humpel, N., N. Owen, and E. Leslie. 2002. Environmental factors associated with adults' participation in physical activity: A review. *American Journal of Preventive Medicine* 22(3): 188–199.

Huon, G., S. Morris, and L. Brown. 1990. Differences between male and female preferences for body size. *Australian Psychologist* 25:314–317.

Institute of Medicine. 2005. *Preventing Childhood Obesity: Health in the Balance.* Washington, D.C.: National Academies Press.

Intergovernmental Panel on Climate Change. Fourth Assessment Report. 2007. http://www.ipcc.ch/.

Janssen, I., W. M. Craig, W. F. Boyce, and W. Pickett. 2004. Associations between overweight and obesity with bullying behaviors in school-aged children. *Pediatrics* 113(5, 1): 1187–1194.

Jee, S. H., J. W. Sull, J. Park, S. Y. Lee, H. Ohrr, E. Guallar, and J. M. Samet. 2006. Body-mass index and mortality in Korean men and women. *New England Journal of Medicine* 355:779–787.

Jeffrey, R., and J. Utter. 2003. The changing environment and population obesity in the United States. *Obesity Research* 11:12S–22S.

Jehn, M., and A. Brewis. 2009. Paradoxical malnutrition in mother-child pairs: Untangling the phenomenon of over- and under-nutrition in underdeveloped economies. *Economics and Human Biology* 7:28–35.

Jenike, M. R. 1996. Activity reduction as an adaptive response to seasonal hunger. *American Journal of Human Biology* 8:517–534.

Joanisse, L., and A. Synnott. 1999. Fighting back: Reactions and resistance to the stigma of obesity. In *Interpreting Weight: The Social Management of Fatness and Thinness*, ed. J. Sobal and D. Maurer, 49–70. New York: Aldine de Gruyter.

Johnston, F., and I. Harkavy. 2009. *The Obesity Culture: Strategies for Change. Public Health and University-Community Partnerships.* London: Smith-Gordon.

Jones, L. R., E. Fries, and S. J. Danish. 2007. Gender and ethnic differences in body image and opposite sex figure preferences of rural adolescents. *Body Image* 4(1): 103–108.

Kaczynski, A. T., L. R. Potwarka, and B. E. Saelens. 2008. Association of park size, distance, and features with physical activity in neighborhood parks. *American Journal of Public Health* 98(8): 1451–1456.

Kahn, R. 2008. Metabolic syndrome—what is the clinical usefulness? *Lancet* 371:1892–1893.

Kana'iaupuni, S., K. Donato, T. Thompson-Colón, and M Stainback. 2005. Counting on kin: Social networks, social support, and child health status. *Social Forces* 83:1137–1164.

Kapoor, S. K., and K. Anand. 2002. Nutritional transition: A public health challenge in developing countries. *Journal of Epidemiology and Community Health* 56:804–805.

Katzmarzyk, P. T., I. Janssen, and C. I. Ardern. 2003. Physical inactivity, excess adiposity, and premature mortality. *Obesity Reviews* 4:257–290.

Keefe, S. E. 1984. Real and ideal extended familism among Mexican-Americans and Anglo-Americans—on the meaning of family ties. *Human Organization* 43(1): 65–70.

Kelly, T., W. Yang, C. S. Chen, K. Reynolds, and J. He. 2008. Global burden of obesity in 2005 and projections to 2030. *International Journal of Obesity* 32(9): 1431–1437.

Kersh, R., and J. Morone. 2002. The politics of obesity: Seven steps to government action. *Health Affairs* 21(6): 142–153.

Khor, G. L., and Z. M. Sharif. 2003. Dual forms of malnutrition in the same households in Malaysia—a case study among Malay rural households. *Asia Pacific Journal of Clinical Nutrition* 12:427–437.

Kiebzak, G. M., L. J. Leamy, L. M. Pierson, R. H. Nord, and Z. Y. Zhang. 2000. Measurement precision of body composition variables using the lunar DPX-L densitometer. *Journal of Clinical Densitometry* 3(1): 35–41.

Kim, S. H., and L. A. Willis. 2007. Talking about obesity: News framing of who is responsible for causing and fixing the problem. *Journal of Health Communication* 12(4): 359–376.

Klein, H., and K. S. Shiffman. 2005. Thin is 'in' and stout is 'out': What animated cartoons tell viewers about body weight. *Eating and Weight Disorders* 10:107–116.

Kleinman, A. 1988. *The Illness Narratives: Suffering, Healing, and the Human Condition.* New York: Basic Books.

Knowler, W. C., D. Pettitt, M. Saad, and P. H. Bennett. 1990. Diabetes mellitus in the Pima Indians: Incidence, risk factors, and pathogenesis. *Diabetes and Metabolism Review* 6:1–27.

Knowler W. C., D. J. Pettitt, P. J. Savage, P. H. Bennett. 1981. Diabetes incidence in Pima Indians: Contributions of obesity and parental diabetes. *American Journal of Epidemiology* 113:144–156.

Komlos, J., and M. Baur. 2004. From the tallest to (one of) the fattest: The enigmatic fate of the size of the American population in the twentieth century. *Economics and Human Biology* 2(1): 57–74.

Kostanski, M., A. Fisher, and E. Gullone. 2004. Current conceptualization of body image dissatisfaction: Have we got it wrong? *Journal of Child Psychology and Psychiatry* 45:1317–1325.

Krieger, N. 1994. Epidemiology and the web of causation: Has anyone seen the spider? *Social Science and Medicine* 39(7): 887–903.

Kriska, A. M., A. Saremi, R. L. Hanson, P. H. Bennett, S. Kobes, D. E. Williams, and W. C. Knowler. 2003. Physical activity, obesity, and the incidence of type 2 diabetes in a high-risk population. *American Journal of Epidemiology* 158:669–675.

Kumanyika, S. K. 1993. Special issues regarding obesity in minority populations. *Annals of Internal Medicine* 119(7 Pt 2): 650–654.

———. 2007. Environmental influences on childhood obesity: Ethnic and cultural influences in context. *Physiology and Behavior* 94(1): 61–70.

———. 2008. Ethnic minorities and weight control research priorities: Where are we now and where do we need to be? *Preventive Medicine* 47(6): 583–586.

Kuzawa, C. W. 1998. Adipose tissue in human infancy and childhood: An evolutionary perspective. *Yearbook of Physical Anthropology* 41:177–209.

Lamb, C. S., L. A. Jackson, P. B. Cassiday, and D. J. Priest. 1993. Body figure preferences of men and women: A comparison of two generations. *Sex Roles* 28:345–358.

Lancaster, J. 1994. Human sexuality, life histories, and evolutionary ecology. In *Sexuality across the Life Course*, ed. A. Rossi, 39–62. Chicago: University of Chicago Press.

Lawrence, R. G. 2004. Framing obesity: The evolution of news discourse on a public health issue. *Harvard International Journal of Press/Politics* 9(3): 56–75.

Lee, S., and A. Brewis. 2009. Children's autonomous food acquisition in Mexican shantytowns. *Ecology of Food and Nutrition* 48(6): 435–456.

Lieberman, L. S. 2003. Dietary, evolutionary, and modernizing influences on the prevalence of type-2 diabetes. *Annual Review of Nutrition* 23:345–377.

Lindquist, C. H., K. D. Reynolds, and M. I. Goran. 1999. Sociocultural determinants of physical activity among children. *Preventive Medicine* 29:305–312.

Lindsay, R. S., and P. H. Bennett. 2001. Type 2 diabetes, the thrifty phenotype—an overview. *British Medical Bulletin* 60:21–32.

Lindsted, K. D., S. Tonstad, and J. W. Kuzma. 1991. Self-report of physical activity and patterns of mortality in Seventh-Day Adventist men. *Journal of Clinical Epidemiology* 44(4–5): 355–364.

Lissau, I., and T. I. Sørensen. 1994. Parental neglect during childhood and increased risk of obesity in young adulthood. *Lancet* 343:324–327.

Littlewood, R. 1995. Psychopathology and personal agency: Modernity, culture change, and eating disorders in South Asian societies. *British Journal of Medical Psychology* 68:45–63.

Lloyd, L. J., S. C. Langley-Evans, and S. McMullen. 2009. Childhood obesity and adult cardiovascular disease risk: A systematic review. *International Journal of Obesity* (advance online publication May 12); doi: 10.1038/ijo.2009.6

Lock, M., and P. Kaufert. 2001. Menopause, local biologies, and cultures of aging. *American Journal of Human Biology* 13(4): 494–504.

Lomnitz, L. 1977. *Networks and Marginality: Life in a Mexican Shantytown*. New York: Academic Press.

Loos, R., and C. Bouchard. 2000. Obesity and cortisol. *Nutrition* 16(10): 924–936.

———. 2008. FTO: The first gene contributing to common forms of obesity. *Obesity Research* 9:246–250.

Loos, R.J.F., et al. 2008. Common variants near *MC4R* are associated with fat mass, weight, and risk of obesity. *Nature Genetics* 40(6): 768–775.

Low, B. S. 2001. Sex, wealth, and fertility: Old rules, new environments. In *Adaptation and Human Behavior: An Anthropological Perspective*, ed. L. Cronk, N. Chagnon, and W. Irons, 323–344. New York: Aldine de Gruyter.

MacKenzie, M. 1985. The pursuit of slenderness and addiction to self-control: An anthropological interpretation of eating disorders. *Nutrition Update* 5:174–194.

Maddox, G. L., K. Back, and V. Liederman. 1965. Overweight as social deviance and disability. *Journal of Health and Social Behaviour* 9(4): 287–298.

Mahmud, N., and N. Crittenden. 2007. A comparative study of body image of Australian and Pakistani young females. *British Journal of Psychology* 98(2): 187–197.

Malcolm, L.W.G. 1925. Note on the seclusion of girls among the Efik at old Calabar. *Man* 25:113–114.

Malina, R. 1996. Regional body composition: Age, sex, and ethnic variation. In *Human Body Composition*, ed. A. F. Roche, S. B. Heymsfield, and T. G. Lohman, 217–255. Champaign, Ill.: Human Kinetics.

Markowitz, D. L., and S. Cosminsky. 2005. Overweight and stunting in migrant Hispanic children in the USA. *Economics and Human Biology* 3(2): 215–240.

Marlowe, F. W., C. L. Apicella, and D. Reed. 2005. Men's preferences for women's profile waist-hip-ratio in two societies. *Evolution and Human Behavior* 26:458–468.

Marlowe, F. W., and A. Wetsman. 2001. Preferred waist-to-hip ratio and ecology. *Personality and Individual Differences* 30(3): 481–489.

Martin, E. 1989. *The Woman in the Body: A Cultural Analysis of Reproduction*. Boston: Beacon Press.

Martin, M. C., and J. W. Gentry. 1997. Stuck in the model trap: The effects of beautiful models in ads on female pre-adolescents and adolescents. *Journal of Advertising* 26(2): 19–34.

Martorell, R., L. K. Khan, M. L. Hughes, and L. M. Grummer-Strawn. 2000. Obesity in women from developing countries. *European Journal of Clinical Nutrition* 54(3): 247–252.

Mascie-Taylor, C.G.N., and R. Goto. 2007. Human variation and body mass index: A review of the universality of BMI cut-offs, gender and urban-rural differences, and secular changes. *Journal of Physiological Anthropology* 26:109–112.

Massara, E. B. 1979. Que Gordita! A study of weight among women in a Puerto Rican community. PhD diss., Bryn Mawr College.

———. 1989. *Que Gordita! A Study of Weight among Women in a Puerto Rican Community.* New York: Community AMS Press.

Maurer, D., and J. Sobal, eds. 1999. *Interpreting Weight: The Social Management of Fatness and Thinness.* New York: Aldine de Gruyter.

McGarvey, S. 1991. Obesity in Samoans and a perspective on its etiology in Polynesians. *American Journal of Clinical Nutrition* 53:1586S–1594S.

———. 1992. Economic modernization and human adaptability perspectives. In *Health and Lifestyle Change*, MASCA, vol. 9, ed. R. Huss-Ashmore, J. Schall, and M. Hediger, 105–112. Philadelphia: University of Pennsylvania Museum of Archeology and Anthropology.

———. 1994. The thrifty gene concept and adiposity studies in biological anthropology. *Journal of the Polynesian Society* 103:29–42.

McGarvey, S., J. Bindon, D. Crews, and D. Schendel. 1989. Modernization and adiposity: Causes and consequences. In *Human Population Biology: A Transdisciplinary Science*, ed. M. Little and J. Haas, 263–279. Oxford: Oxford University Press.

McGarvey, S., P. Levinson, L. Bausserman, D. Galanis, and C. Hornick. 1993. Population change in adult obesity and blood lipids in American Samoa from 1976–78 to 1990. *American Journal of Human Biology* 5:17–30.

McLaren, L. 2007. Socioeconomic status and obesity. *Epidemiological Reviews* 29:29–48.

McNeely, M. J., and E. J. Boyko. 2004. Type 2 diabetes prevalence in Asian Americans: Results of a national health survey. *Diabetes Care* 27(1): 66–69.

Mendez, M. A., C. A. Monteiro, and B. M. Popkin. 2005. Overweight now exceeds underweight among women in most developing countries! *American Journal of Clinical Nutrition* 81:714–721.

Mendez, M. A., and B. M. Popkin. 2004. Globalization, urbanization, and nutritional change in the developing world. In *FAO. Globalization of Food Systems in Developing Countries: Impact on Food Security and Nutrition*, 55–80. FAO Food and Nutrition Paper No. 83. Rome: FAO.

Menjivar, C. 2000. *Fragmented Ties: Salvadoran Immigrant Networks in America.* Berkeley: University of California Press.

Mennis, J. L., and L. Jordan. 2005. The distribution of environmental equity: Exploring spatial nonstationarity in multivariate models of air toxic releases. *Annals of the Association of American Geographers* 95(2): 249–268.

Mikkelsen, L., and S. Chemini. 2007. *The Links between Neighborhood Food Environment and Childhood Nutrition.* Princeton, N.J.: Robert Wood Johnson Foundation.

Miller, E., and J. Halberstadt. 2005. Media consumption, body image, and thin ideals in New Zealand men and women. *New Zealand Journal of Psychology* 34(3): 189–195.

Millman, M. 1980. *Such a Pretty Face: Being Fat in America.* New York: Norton.

Milton, K. 2000. Back to basics: Why foods of wild primates have relevance for modern human health. *Nutrition* 16(7–8): 480–483.

——. 2002. Hunter-gatherer diets: Wild foods signal relief from diseases of affluence. In *Human Diet: Its Origins and Evolution*, ed. P. S. Ungar and M. F. Teaford, 111–122. Westport, Conn.: Bergin and Garvey.

Mintz, L. B., and S. K. Kashubeck. 1999. Body-image and disordered eating among Asian American and Caucasian college students. *Psychology of Women Quarterly* 23:781–796.

Moffat, T., and T. Galloway. 2007. Adverse environments: Investigating local variation in child growth and health. *American Journal of Human Biology* 19(5): 676–683.

Mokdad, A. H., E. S. Ford, B. A. Bowman, W. H. Dietz, F. Vinicor, V. S. Bales, and J. S. Marks. 2003. Prevalence of obesity, diabetes, and obesity-related health factors, 2001. *Journal of the American Medical Association* 289(1): 76–79.

Monteiro, C. A., W. L. Conde, and B. M. Popkin. 2004. The burden of disease from undernutrition and overnutrition in countries undergoing rapid nutrition transition: A view from Brazil. *American Journal of Public Health* 94:433–434.

Monteiro, C. A., E. C. Moura, W. L. Conde, and B. M. Popkin. 2004. Socioeconomic status and obesity in adult populations of developing countries: A review. *Bulletin of the World Health Organization* 82(12): 891–979.

Morello-Frosch, R., and R. Lopez. 2006. The riskscape and the color line: Examining the role of segregation in environmental health disparities. *Environmental Research* 102(2): 181–196.

Moreno, A. B., and M. H. Thelen. 1993. A preliminary prevention program for eating disorders in a junior high school population. *Journal of Youth and Adolescence* 22:109–124.

Morland, K., A. Diez Roux, and S. Wing. 2002. The contextual effect of the local food environment on residents' diets: The Atherosclerosis Risk in Communities Study. *American Journal of Public Health* 92(11): 1761–1767.

——. 2006. Supermarkets, other food stores, and obesity. *American Journal of Preventive Medicine* 30:333–339.

Murphy, J., and S. McGarvey. 1994. Modernization in the Samoas and children's reactivity: A pilot study. *Psychosomatic Medicine* 56:395–400.

Musaiger, A. O., N. E. Shahbeek, and M. Al-Mannai. 2004. The role of social factors and weight status in ideal body-shape preferences as perceived by Arab women. *Journal of Biosocial Science* 36(6): 699–707.

Neel, J. V. 1962. Diabetes mellitus: A "thrifty" genotype rendered detrimental by "progress"? *American Journal of Human Genetics* 14:353–362.

Nelson, L., T. Pettijohn, and J. Galak. 2007. Mate preferences in social cognitive context: When environmental and personal change leads to predictable cross-cultural variation. In *Body Beautiful: Evolutionary and Sociocultural Perspectives*, ed. V. Swami and A. Furnham, 85–206. New York: Palgrave Macmillan.

Newell, B., K. Proust, R. Dyball, and P. McManus. 2007. Seeing obesity as a systems problem. *NSW Public Health Bulletin* 18(11–12): 214–218.

New Zealand Ministry of Health. 2008. *A Portrait of Health: Key Results of the 2006/07 New Zealand Health Survey*. Wellington, New Zealand: Ministry of Health.

NHANES [National Health and Nutrition Examination Survey]. 2007. http://www.cdc.gov/nchs/nhanes.htm.

Nichter, M. 2000. *Fat Talk: What Girls and Their Parents Say about Dieting*. Cambridge, Mass.: Harvard University Press.

Nicolau, M., C. Doak, R. Dam, K. Hosper, J. Seidell, and K. Stronks. 2008. Body size preference and body weight perception among two migrant groups of non-Western origin. *Public Health Nutrition* 11(12): 1332–1341.

NIH [National Institutes of Health]. Department of Health and Human Services. 2008. Innovative computational and statistical methodologies for the design and analysis of multilevel studies on childhood obesity. Part I: Overview Information. http://grants.nih.gov/grants/guide/rfa-files/RFA-HD-08-023.html.

NIH [National Institutes of Health] and NHLBI [National Heart, Lung, and Blood Institute]. 1998. Clinical guidelines on the identification, evaluation, and treatment of overweight and obesity in adults—the evidence report. *Obesity Research* 6(2): 1S–209S.

Nord, M., M. Andrews, and S. Carlson. 2008. *Household Food Security in the United States, 2007.* Economic Research Report No. (ERR-66). Washington, D.C.: U.S. Department of Agriculture.

Norgan, N. G. 1994. Population differences in body composition in relation to the body mass index. *European Journal of Clinical Nutrition* 48(3): S10–S27.

Norgan, N. G., and P.R.M. Jones. 1995. The effect of standardising the body mass index for relative sitting height. *International Journal of Obesity Related Metabolic Disorders* 19:206–208.

Norman, R. A., P. A. Tataranni, R. Pratley, D. B. Thompson, R. L. Hanson, M. Prochazka, L. Baier, M. G. Ehm, H. Sakul, T. Foroud, W. T. Garvey, D. Burns, W. C. Knowler, P. H. Bennett, C. Bogardus, and E. Ravussin. 1998. Autosomal genomic scan for loci linked to obesity and energy metabolism in Pima Indians. *American Journal of Human Genetics* 62(3): 659–668.

Oakes, M. J. 2008. Invited commentary: Rescuing Robinson Crusoe. *American Journal of Epidemiology* 168:9–12.

Oakes, M. J., and P. H. Rossi. 2003. The measurement of SES in health research: Current practice and steps toward a new approach. *Social Science and Medicine* 56(4): 769–784.

Ogden, C. L., M. D. Carroll, L. R. Curtin, M. A. McDowell, C. J. Tabak, and K. M. Flegal. 2006. Prevalence of overweight and obesity in the United States, 1999–2004. *Journal of the American Medical Association* 295(13): 1549–1555.

Ogden, J., and K. Mundray. 1996. The effect of the media on body satisfaction: The role of gender and size. *European Eating Disorders Review* 4:171–182.

Olshansky, S. J., D. Passaro, R. Hershow, J. Layden, B. A. Carnes, J. Brody, L. Hayflick, R. N. Butler, D. B. Allison, and D. S. Ludwig. 2005. A potential decline in life expectancy in the United States in the 21st century. *New England Journal of Medicine* 352:1138–1145.

Olvera-Ezzell, N., T. G. Power, and J. H. Cousins. 1990. Maternal socialization of children's eating habits: Strategies used by obese Mexican-American mothers. *Child Development* 61(2): 395.

Omer, I., and U. Or. 2005. Distributive environmental justice in the city: Differential access in two mixed Israeli cities. *Tijdschrift voor Economische en Sociale Geografie* 96(4): 433–443.

Ono, T., R. Guthold, and K. Strong. 2005. *WHO Comparable Estimates.* Geneva: World Health Organization.

Orsini, N., R. Bellocco, M. Bottai, M. Pagano, K. Michaelsson, and A. Wolk. 2008. Combined effects of obesity and physical activity in predicting mortality among men. *Journal of Internal Medicine* 264(5): 442–451.

Parker, S., M. Nichter, N. Vukovic, C. Sims, and C. Ritenbaugh. 1995. Body image and weight concerns among African American and White adolescent females: Differences that make a difference. *Human Organization* 54:103–114.

Pastor, M., R. Morello-Frosch, and J. L. Sadd. 2005. The air is always cleaner on the other side: Race, space, and ambient air toxics exposures in California. *Journal of Urban Affairs* 27:127–148.

Pelletier, D. 2006. Theoretical considerations related to cutoff points. *Food and Nutrition Bulletin* 27: S224–S236.

Pellow, D. N., and R. J. Brulle. 2006. *Power, Justice, and the Environment: A Critical Appraisal of the Environmental Justice Movement.* Cambridge, Mass.: MIT Press.

Perry, A. C., E. B. Rosenblatt, and X. Wang. 2004. Physical, behavioral, and body image characteristics in a tri-racial group of adolescent girls. *Obesity Research* 12:1670–1679.

Pettijohn, T. F., and A. Tesser. 1999. Popularity in environmental context: Facial feature assessment of American movie actresses. *Media Psychology* 1:229–247.

Pike, I. L., and C. Patil. 2006. Understanding women's burdens: Preliminary findings on psychosocial health among Datoga and Iraqw women of northern Tanzania. *Culture, Medicine, and Psychiatry* 30:299–330.

Pike, M., and A. Borovoy. 2004. The rise of eating disorders in Japan: Issues of culture and limitations of the model of "Westernization." *Culture, Medicine, and Psychiatry* 28(4): 493–531.

Pollan, M. 2007. *The Omnivore's Dilemma*. New York: Penguin Press.

Pool, R. 2000. *Fat: Fighting the Obesity Epidemic*. New York: Oxford University Press.

Popenoe, R. 2004. *Feeding Desire: Fatness, Beauty, and Sexuality among a Saharan People*. London and New York: Routledge.

Popkin, B. M. 1994. The nutrition transition in low-income countries: An emerging crisis. *Nutritional Reviews* 52(9): 285–298.

———. 2008. Will China's nutrition transition overwhelm its health care system and slow economic growth? *Health Affairs* 27:1064–1076.

———. 2009. *The World Is Fat: The Fads, Trends, Policies, and Products That Are Fattening the Human Race*. New York: Avery.

Popkin, B. M., and J. R. Udry. 1998. Adolescent obesity increases significantly in second and third generation U.S. immigrants: The National Longitudinal Study of Adolescent Health. *Journal of Nutrition* 128(4): 701–706.

Poston, W.S.C., and J. P. Foreyt. 1999. Obesity is an environmental issue. *Atherosclerosis* 146:201–209.

Powell, L., M. Auld, F. Chaloupka, P. O'Malley, and L. Johnston. 2007. Associations between access to food stores and adolescent body mass index. *American Journal of Preventive Medicine* 33:S301–S307.

Powell, L., S. Slater, D. Mirtcheva, Y. Bao, and F. J. Chaloupka. 2007. Food store availability and neighborhood characteristics in the United States. *American Journal of Preventive Medicine* 44:189–195.

Prentice, A. M. 2006. The emerging epidemic of obesity in developing countries. *International Journal of Epidemiology* 35:24–30.

Prentice, A. M., and T. J. Cole. 1994. Seasonal changes in growth and energy status in the Third World. *Proceedings of the Nutrition Society* 53:509–519.

Preston, S. H. 2005. Deadweight? *New England Journal of Medicine* 352:1135–1137.

Puhl, R., and K. D. Brownell. 2001. Bias, discrimination, and obesity. *Obesity Research* 9:788–805.

———. 2006. Confronting and coping with weight stigma: An investigation of overweight and obese individuals. *Obesity Research* 14:1802–1815.

Puhl, R. M., and C. A. Heuer. 2009. The stigma of obesity: A review and update. *Obesity Research* 17(5): 941–964.

Rand, C.S.W., and A.M.C. McGregor. 1990. Morbidly obese patients' perceptions of social discrimination before and after surgery for obesity. *Southern Medical Journal* 83:1390–1395.

Rand, C.S.W., and B. A. Wright. 2000. Continuity and change in the evaluation of ideal and acceptable body sizes across a wide age span. *International Journal of Eating Disorders* 28:90–100.

Raphaël, D., H. Delisle, and C. Vilgrain. 2005. Households with undernourished children and overweight mothers: Is this a concern for Haiti? *Ecology of Food and Nutrition* 44(2): 147–165.

Raphael, F., and J. Lacey. 1992. Sociocultural aspects of eating disorders. *Annals of Medicine* 24:293–296.

Reischer, E., and K. Koo. 2004. The body beautiful: Symbolism and agency in the social world. *Annual Review of Anthropology* 33:297–317.

Rguibi, M., and R. Belahsen. 2006. Body size preferences and sociocultural influences on attitudes towards obesity among Moroccan Sahraoui women. *Body Image* 3(4): 395–400.

Ritenbaugh, C. 1981. A clinal view of diabetes. *Anthropology UCLA* 7:183–188.

———. 1982. Obesity as a culture-bound syndrome. *Culture Medical Psychiatry* 6:347–364.

Roberts, A., T. F. Cash, A. Feingold, and B. T. Johnson. 2006. Are Black-White differences in females' body dissatisfaction decreasing? A meta-analytic review. *Journal of Consulting and Clinical Psychology* 74(6): 1121–1131.

Robinson, T., M. Callister, and T. Jankowski. 2008. Portrayal of body weight on children's television sitcoms: A content analysis. *Body Image* 5(2): 141–151.

Robison, J. 2006. Health at every size. *Absolute Advantage* 5(3): 8–13.

Robison, J., S. L. Hoerr, K. A. Petersmarck, and J. V. Anderson. 1995. Redefining success in obesity intervention: The new paradigm. *Journal of the American Dietetic Association* 95:422–423.

Rodin, J., L. Silberstein, and R. Striegel-Moore. 1985. Women and weight: A normative discontent. In *Psychology and Gender: Nebraska Symposium on Motivation, 1984*, ed. T. B. Sonderegger, 267–307. Lincoln: University of Nebraska Press.

Roemmich, J. N., L. H. Epstein, S. Raja, L. Yin, J. Robinson, and D. Winiewicz. 2006. Association of access to parks and recreational facilities with the physical activity of young children. *Journal of Preventive Medicine* 43:437–441.

Rogge, M. E., and T. Combs-Orme. 2003. Protecting children from chemical exposure: Social work and U.S. social welfare policy. *Social Work* 48(4): 439–450.

Rolland-Cachera, M. F., T. J. Sempé, J. Tichet, C. Rossignol, and A. Charraud. 1991. Body mass index variations: Centiles from birth to 87 years. *European Journal of Clinical Nutrition* 45(1): 13–21.

Romero-Corral, A., V. M. Montori, V. K. Somers, J. Korinek, R. J. Thomas, T. G. Allison, F. Mookadam, and F. López-Jiménez. 2006. Association of bodyweight with total mortality and with cardiovascular events in coronary artery disease: A systematic review of cohort studies. *Lancet* 368:666–678.

Romero-Corral, A., V. K. Somers, J. Sierra-Johnson, R. J. Thomas, M. L. Collazo-Clavell, J. Korinek, T. G. Allison, J. A. Batsis, F. H. Sert-Kuniyoshi, and F. Lopez-Jimenez. 2008. Accuracy of body mass index in diagnosing obesity in the adult general population. *International Journal of Obesity* 32:959–966.

Ronai, C. R. 1997. Discursive constraint in the narrated identities of childhood sex abuse survivors. In *Everyday Sexism in the Third Millennium*, ed. C. R. Ronai, B. A. Zsembik, and J. R. Feagin, 123–136. New York: Routledge.

Roscoe, J. 1923. The Negro-Hamitic people of Uganda. *Scottish Geographical Journal* 39(3): 145–159.

Rose, D. 2007. Food stamps, the Thrifty Food Plan, and meal preparation: The importance of the time dimension for US nutrition policy. *Journal of Nutrition Education and Behavior* 39(4): 226–232.

Rose, D., and R. Richards. 2004. Food store access and household fruit and vegetable use among participants in the U.S. Food Stamp Program. *Public Health Nutrition* 7:1081–1088.

Roth, J. 2009a. Evolutionary speculation about tuberculosis and the metabolic and inflammatory processes of obesity. *Journal of the American Medical Association* 301(24): 2586–2588.

Roth, J. 2009b. Tuberculosis and the inflammatory processes of obesity in human evolu-tion—Reply. *Journal of the American Medical Association* 302(16): 1754–1755.

Rozin, P., and A. Fallon. 1988. Body image, attitudes to weight, and misperceptions of figure preferences of the opposite sex: A comparison of men and women in two generations. *Journal of Abnormal Psychology* 97:342–345.

Rozin, P., S. Trachtenberg, and A. B. Cohen. 2001. Stability of body image and body image dissatisfaction in American college students over about the last 15 years. *Appetite* 37(3): 245–248.

Rubin, N., C. Shmilovitz, and M. Weiss. 1993. From fat to thin: Informal rites affirming iden-tity change. *Symbolic Interaction* 16:1–17.

Rucker, C. E., and T. F. Cash. 1992. Body images, body-size perceptions, and eating behaviors among African American and White college women. *International Journal of Eating Disorders* 12:291–299.

Ryan, A., A. Roche, and R. Kuczmarski. 1999. Weight, stature, and body mass index data for Mexican Americans from the third National Health and Nutrition Examination Survey (NHANES III, 1988–1994). *American Journal of Human Biology* 11:673–786.

Saelens, B. E., J. F. Sallis, J. B. Black, and D. Chen. 2003. Neighborhood-based differences in physical activity: An environment scale evaluation. *American Journal of Public Health* 93(9): 1552–1558.

Safir, M. P., S. Flaisher-Kellner, and A. Rosenmann. 2005. When gender differences surpass cultural difference in personal satisfaction with body shape in Israel. *Sex Roles* 52(5–6): 369–378.

Saito, S. 1995. *1993 National Nutrition Survey Main Report*. Suva, Fiji: National Food and Nutrition Committee.

Sallis, J. F., and K. Glanz. 2006. The role of built environments in physical activity, eating, and obesity in childhood. *Future of Children* 16(1): 89–108.

Sanchez-Johnsen, L. A. P., M. L. Fitzgibbon, Z. Martinovich, M. R. Stolley, A. R. Dyer, and L. Van Horn. 2004. Ethnic differences in correlates of obesity between Latin-American and Black women. *Obesity Research* 12:652–660.

Sanchez-Vaznaugh, E. V., I. Kawachi, S. V. Subramanian, B. N. Sánchez, and D. Acevedo-Garcia. 2008. Differential effect of birthplace and length of residence on body mass index (BMI) by education, gender and race/ethnicity. *Social Science and Medicine* 67(8): 1300–1310.

Sanders, N. M., and C. J. Heiss. 1998. A comparison of body image and eating attitudes in Asian and Caucasian college women. *Eating Disorders: Treatment and Prevention* 6:15–27.

Sarlio-Lähteenkorva, S. 2001. Weight loss and quality of life among obese people. *Social Indicators Research* 54: 329–54.

Scagliusi, F. B., M. Alvarenga, V. O. Polaco, T. A. Cordás, G. K. de Oliveira Queiroz, D. Coelho, S. T. Philippi, and A. H. Lancha Jr. 2006. Concurrent and discriminant validity of the Stunkard's figure rating scale adapted into Portuguese. *Appetite* 47(1): 77–82.

Scharoun-Lee, M., L. S. Adair, J. S. Kaufman, and P. Gordon-Larsen. 2009. Obesity, race/eth-nicity, and the multiple dimensions of socioeconomic status during the transition to adulthood: A factor analysis approach. *Social Science and Medicine* 68(4): 708–716.

Schell, L. M. 1992. Risk focusing: An example of biocultural interaction. In *Health and Lifestyle Change*, ed. R. Huss-Ashmore, J. Schall, and M. Hediger, 137–144. Philadelphia: University of Pennsylvania Press.

———. 1997. Culture as a stressor: A revised model of biocultural interaction. *American Journal of Physical Anthropology* 102(1): 67–77.

———. 2003. Polluted environments as extreme environments: Evidence for effects on growth. In *Human Growth from Conception to Maturity*, ed. G. Gilli, L. Benso, and L. Schell, 249–261. London: Smith-Gordon.

Schell, L. M., and P. D. Magnus. 2007. Is there an elephant in the room? Addressing rival approaches to the interpretation of growth perturbations and small size. *American Journal of Human Biology* 19(5): 606–614.

Schell, L. M., J. Ravenscroft, M. Cole, A. Jacobs, and J. Newman. 2005. Health disparities and toxicant exposure of Akwesasne Mohawk young adults: A partnership approach to research. *Environmental Health Perspectives* 113(12): 1826–1832.

Schwartz, M. B., L. R. Vartanian, B. A. Nosek, and K. D. Brownell. 2006. The influence of one's own body weight on implicit and explicit anti-fat bias. *Obesity* 14:440–447.

Scott, I., G. Bentley, M. Tovee, F. U. Ahamed, and K. Magid. 2007. An evolutionary perspective on male preferences for female body shape. In *The Body Beautiful: Evolutionary and Sociocultural Perspectives*, ed. V. Swami and A. Furnham, 56–87. New York: Palgrave Macmillan.

Sharkey, J., and S. Horel. 2008. Neighborhood socioeconomic deprivation and minority composition are associated with better potential spatial access to the ground-truthed food environment in a large rural area. *Journal of Nutrition* 138:620–627.

Sharps, M. J., J. L. Sharps-Price, and J. Hanson. 2001. Body image preference in the United States and rural Thailand: An exploratory study. *Journal of Psychology* 135(5): 518–526.

Shaw, J., and G. Waller. 1995. The media's impact on body image: Implications for prevention and treatment. *Journal of Treatment and Prevention* 3(2): 115–123.

Sherraden, M., and R. Barrera. 1996. Poverty, family support, and well-being of infants: Mexican immigrant women and childbearing. *Journal of Sociology and Social Welfare* 23:27–54.

Shih, M. Y., and C. Kubo. 2002. Body shape preference and body satisfaction in Taiwanese college students. *Psychiatry Research* 111(2–3): 215–228.

Shulz, L. O., P. Bennett, E. Ravussin, J. Kidd, K. Kidd, J. Esparza, and M. E. Valencia. 2006. Effects of traditional and western environments on prevalence of type 2 diabetes in Pima Indians in Mexico and the U.S. *Diabetes Care* 29(8): 1866–1871.

Siegel, K., H. Lune, and I. H. Meyer. 1998. Stigma management among gay/bisexual men with HIV/AIDS. *Qualitative Sociology* 21(1): 3–24.

Simeon, D. T., R. D. Rattan, K. Panchoo, K. V. Kungeesingh, A. C. Ali, and P. S. Abdool. 2003. Body image of adolescents in a multi-ethnic Caribbean population. *European Journal of Clinical Nutrition* 57:157–162.

Simmons, R. G., and M. Rosenberg. 1971. Functions of children's perceptions of the stratification system. *American Sociological Review* 36:235–249.

Simon, G. E., M. Von Korff, K. Saunders, D. L. Miglioretti, P. K. Crane, G. van Belle, and R. C. Kessler. 2006. Association between obesity and psychiatric disorders in the U.S. adult population. *Archives of General Psychiatry* 63:824–830.

Singer, M., and H. Baer. 2007. *Introducing Medical Anthropology: A Discipline in Action.* Lanham, Md.: Altamira Press.

Singh, D. 1993. Body shape and women's attractiveness: The critical role of waist–hip ratio. *Human Nature* 4:297–321.

———. 1994. Is thin really beautiful and good? Relationship between physical attractiveness and waist-to-hip ratio. *Personality and Individual Differences* 16:123–132.

Singh, D., and R. Young. 1995. Body weight, WHR, breasts and hips: Role in judgments of female attractiveness and desirability for relationships. *Ethology and Sociobiology* 16:483–507.

Sjoberg, R. L., K. W. Nilsson, and J. Leppert. 2005. Obesity, shame, and depression in school-aged children: A population-based study. *Pediatrics* 116(3): e389–e392.

Sloane, D. C., A. L. Diamant, L. B. Lewis, A. K. Yancey, G. Flynn, L. M. Nascimento, W. J. McCarthy, J. J. Guinyard, M. R. Cousineau, and the REACH Coalition of the African

American Building a Legacy of Health Project. 2003. Improving the nutritional resource environment for healthy living through community-based participatory research. *Journal of General Internal Medicine* 18:568–575.

Smith, A. R., and T. E. Joiner. 2008. Examining body image discrepancies and perceived weight status in adult Japanese women. *Eating Behaviors* 9:513–515.

Smith, C., K. Schmoll, J. Konik, and S. Oberlander. 2007. Carrying weight for the world: Influence of weight descriptors on judgments of large-sized women. *Journal of Applied Social Psychology* 37:989–1006.

Smith, C. J., R. G. Nelson, S. A. Hardy, E. M. Manahan, P. H. Bennett, and W. C. Knowler. 1996. Survey of the diet of Pima Indians using quantitative food frequency assessment and 24-hour recall: Diabetic Renal Disease Study. *Journal of American Dietetic Association* 96:778–784.

Smith, D., and C. Cogswell. 1994. A Cross-cultural perspective on adolescent girls' body perception. *Perceptual and Motor Skills* 78:744–746.

Smith, D. E., J. K. Thompson, J. M. Raczynski, and J. E. Hilner. 1999. Body image among men and women in a biracial cohort: The CARDIA study. *International Journal of Eating Disorders* 25:71–82.

Smith, K. R., B. B. Brown, I. Yamada, L. Kowalwski-Jones, C. Zick, and J. X. Fan. 2008. Walkability and body mass index: Density, design, and new diversity measures. *American Journal of Preventive Medicine* 35(3): 237–244.

Smith-Morris, C. 2004. Reducing diabetes in Indian country: Lessons from the three domains influencing Pima diabetes. *Human Organization* 63(1): 34–46.

———. 2006. *Diabetes among the Pima: Stories of Survival.* Tucson: University of Arizona Press.

Smoyer-Tomic, K. E., J. C. Spence, K. D. Raine, C. Amrhein, N. Cameron, V. Yasenovskiy, N. Cutumisu, E. Hemphill, and J. Healy. 2008. The association between neighborhood socioeconomic status and exposure to supermarkets and fast food outlets. *Health and Place* 12:740–754.

Snijder, M. B., R. M. van Dam, M. Visser, and J. C. Seidell. 2006. What aspects of body fat are particularly hazardous and how do we measure them? *International Journal of Epidemiology* 35:83–92.

Snyder, L. B., and M. A. Hamilton. 2002. Meta-analysis of U.S. health campaign effects on behavior: Emphasize enforcement, exposure, and new information, and beware the secular trend. In *Public Health Communication: Evidence for Behavior Change*, ed. R. Hornik, 357–383. Hillsdale, N.J.: Lawrence Erlbaum Associates.

Sobal, J. 1995. The medicalization and demedicalization of obesity. In *Eating Agendas: Food and Nutrition as Social Problems*, ed. D. Maurer and J. Sobal, 67–90. New York: Aldine de Gruyter.

———. 1999. The size acceptance movement and the social construction of body weight. In *Interpreting Weight: The Social Management of Fatness and Thinness*, ed. J. Sobal and D. Maurer, 231–249. New York: Aldine de Gruyter.

———. 2001. Commentary: Globalization and the epidemiology of obesity. *International Journal of Epidemiology* 30:1136–1137.

Sobal, J., and A. J. Stunkard. 1989. Socioeconomic status and obesity: A review of the literature. *Psychological Bulletin* 105(2): 260–275.

Sobo, E. 1993. Bodies, kin, and flow: Family planning in rural Jamaica. *Medical Anthropology Quarterly* 7(1): 50–73.

———. 1994. The sweetness of fat: Health, procreation, and sociability in rural Jamaica. In *Many Mirrors: Body Image and Social Meaning*, ed. N. Sault, 132–154. New Brunswick, N.J.: Rutgers University Press.

———. 2008. *Health Services Research: A Practical Field Guide*. Walnut Creek, Calif.: Left Coast Press.

Stevens, C., and M. Tiggemann. 1998. Women's body figure preferences across the life span. *Journal of Genetic Psychology* 159(1): 94–102.

Stevens, J., J. E. McClain, and K. P. Truesdale. 2006. Commentary: Obesity claims and controversies. *International Journal of Epidemiology* 35(1): 77–78.

Streeter, S. A., and D. H. McBurney. 2003. Waist-hip ratio and attractiveness: New evidence and a critique of a critical test. *Evolution and Human Behavior* 24:88–98.

Striegel-Moore, R. H., G. B. Schreiber, K. M. Pike, D. E. Wilfley, and J. Rodin. 1995. Drive for thinness in black and white preadolescent girls. *International Journal of Eating Disorders* 18:59–69.

Stunkard, A. J. 2000. Old and new scales for the assessment of body image. *Perceptual and Motor Skills* 90(3): 930.

Stunkard, A. J., and J. Sobal. 1995. Psychosocial consequences of obesity. In *Eating Disorders and Obesity*, ed. K. D. Brownell and C. G. Fairburn, 417–421. New York: Guilford Press.

Stunkard, A. J., T. Sorensen, and F. Schulsinger. 1983. Use of the Danish adoption register for the study of obesity and thinness. In *Genetics of Neurological and Psychiatric Disorder*, ed. S. S. Kety, L. P. Rowland, R. L. Sidman, and S. W. Matthysse, 115–120. New York: Raven Press.

Sturm, R., and K. Wells. 2001. Does obesity contribute as much to morbidity as poverty and smoking? *Public Health* 115:229–295.

Sugiyama, L. S. 2004. Is beauty in the context-sensitive adaptations of the beholder?: Shiwiar use of waist-to-hip ratio in assessments of female mate value. *Evolution and Human Behavior* 25(1): 52–63.

Sullivan, L. 1921. *A Contribution to Samoan Somatology*. Honolulu: BP Bishop Museum.

Sundquist, J., and M. Winkleby. 2000. Country of birth, acculturation status, and abdominal obesity in a national sample of Mexican-American women and men. *International Journal of Epidemiology* 29(3): 470–477.

Super, C. M., and S. Harkness. 1982. The infant's niche in rural Kenya and metropolitan America. In *Cross-Cultural Research at Issue*, ed. L. L. Adler, 47–56. New York: Academic Press.

Swami, V., N. Antonakopoulos, M. J. Tovée, and A. Furnham. 2006. A critical test of the waist-to-hip ratio hypothesis of female physical attractiveness in Britain and Greece. *Sex Roles* 54:201–211.

Swami, V, and A. Furnham. 2008. *The Body Beautiful: Evolutionary and Sociocultural Perspectives*. New York: Palgrave Macmillan.

Swami, V., F. Neto, M. J. Tovée, and A. Furnham. 2007. Preference for female body weight and shape in three European countries. *European Psychologist* 12:220–227.

Swami, V., and M. J. Tovée. 2005. Female physical attractiveness in Britain and Malaysia: A cross-cultural study. *Body Image* 2:115–128.

———. 2007. Perceptions of female body weight and shape among indigenous and urban Europeans. *Scandinavian Journal of Psychology* 48:43–50.

Swinburn B., H. Amosa, and A. Bell. 1997. The Ola Fa'autauta project: The process of developing a church-based health promotion programme. *Pacific Health Dialog* 4:20–25.

Swinburn, B., P. Craig, B. Strauss, and R. Daniel. 1995. Body mass index: Is it an appropriate measure of obesity in Polynesians? *Asia Pacific Journal of Clinical Nutrition* 4:367.

Swinburn B. P, S. J. Ley, H. E. Carmichael, and L. D. Plank. 1999. Body size and composition in Polynesians. *International Journal of Obesity* 3(11): 1178–1183.

Szkupinski Quiroga, S., A. Brewis, and A. Wutich. 2008. New multimodal techniques in combating childhood obesity and diabetes. Paper presented at the annual meeting of the Society for Applied Anthropology, Memphis, Tennessee.

Thomas, R. B. 1998. The evolution of human adaptability paradigms: Toward a biology of poverty. In *Building a New Biocultural Synthesis: Political-Economic Perspectives on Human Biology*, ed. A. Goodman and T. Leatherman, 43–73. Ann Arbor: University of Michigan Press.

Thompson, J. K. 1996. *Body Image, Eating Disorders, and Obesity: An Integrative Guide for Assessment and Treatment*. Washington, D.C.: American Psychological Association.

Tiggemann, M., and E. Ruutel. 2001. A cross-cultural comparison of body dissatisfaction in Estonian and Australian young adults and its relationship with media exposure. *Journal of Cross-Cultural Psychology* 32(6): 736–774.

Timperio, A., J. Salmon, A. Telford, and D. Crawford. 2005. Perceptions of local neighborhood environments and their relationship to childhood overweight and obesity. *International Journal of Obesity* 29(2): 170–175.

Tomasello, M. 2008. *Origins of Human Communication*. Cambridge, Mass.: MIT Press.

Tovée, M. J., A. Furnham, and V. Swami. 2007. Healthy body equals beautiful body? Changing perceptions of health and attractiveness with shifting socioeconomic status. In *The Body Beautiful: Evolutionary and Socio-cultural Perspectives*, ed. A. Furnham and V. Swami, 108–128. New York: Palgrave Macmillan.

Tovée, M. J., P. J. Hancock, S. Mahmoodi, B. R. Singleton, and P. L. Cornelissen. 2002. Human female attractiveness: Waveform analysis of body shape. *Proceedings of the Royal Society B: Biological Sciences* 269(1506): 2205–2213.

Tovée, M. J., D. Maisey, J. Emery, and P. Cornelissen. 1999. Visual cues to female physical attractiveness. *Proceedings of the Royal Society B: Biological Sciences* 266:211–218.

Tovée, M. J., and V. Swami. 2005. Female attractiveness in Britain and Malaysia: A cross-cultural study. *Body Image* 2:115–128.

Tovée, M. J., V. Swami, A. Furnham, and R. Mangalparsad. 2006. Changing perceptions of attractiveness as observers are exposed to a different culture. *Evolution and Human Behavior* 27(6): 443–456.

Trail, W. B. 2006. Trends towards overweight in lower- and middle-income countries: some causes and economic policy options. http://www.fao.org/docrep/009/a0442e/a0442 eox.htm.

Trostle, J. 2005. *Epidemiology and Culture*. New York: Cambridge University Press.

Tsai, C. Y., S. L. Hoerr, and W. O. Song. 1998. Dieting behavior of Asian college women attending a U.S. university. *Journal of American College Health* 46(4): 163–170.

Tufano, J. T., and B. Karras. 2005. Mobile ehealth interventions for obesity: A timely opportunity to leverage convergence trends. *Journal of Medical Internet Research* 7(5): e58.

Turner, B. 1984. *The Body in Society*. Oxford: Basil Blackwell.

Ulijaszek, S. 2005. Modernisation, migration, and nutritional health of Pacific Island populations. *Environmental Sciences* 12(3): 167–176.

———. 2005. Obesity in Pacific nations. *Human Ecology* 13:23–28.

USDA [U.S. Department of Agriculture] Forest Service. 2006. National survey on recreation and the environment. Athens, Ga.: USDA Forest Service, Southern Research Station.

Valente, T. W. 1995. *Network Models of Diffusion of Innovations*. Cresskill, N.J.: Hampton Press.

VanDiver, T. A. 1997. Relationship of mothers' perceptions and behavior to the duration of breastfeeding. *Psychological Reports* 80:1375–1384.

Wachs, T. D. 2008. Multiple influences on children's nutritional deficiencies: A systems perspective. *Physiology and Behavior* 94(1): 48–60.

Wadden, T., L. Womble, A. Stunkard, and D. Anderson. 2002. Psychosocial consequences of obesity and weight loss. In *Handbook of Obesity Treatment*, ed. T. Wadden and A. Stunkard, 144–169. New York: Guildford Press.

Walden, K. 1985. The road to fat city: An interpretation of the development of weight consciousness in Western society. *Historical Reflections* 12:331–373.

Walsh, B. T., and M. J. Devlin. 1998. Eating disorders: Progress and problems. *Science* 280(5368): 1387–1390.

Wang, Y. 2001. Cross-national comparison of childhood obesity: The epidemic and the relationships between obesity and socioeconomic status. *International Journal of Epidemiology* 30:1129–1136.

Wang, Y., and M. Beydoun. 2007. The obesity epidemic in the United States—gender, age, socioeconomic, racial/ethnic, and geographic characteristics: A systematic review and meta-regression analysis. *Epidemiology Review* 29:6–28.

Wang, Y., and Q. Zhang. 2006. Are low-socioeconomic status American children and adolescents at increased risk of obesity? Trends in the association between overweight and family income between 1971 and 2002. *American Journal of Clinical Nutrition* 84:707–716.

Wardle, J., R. Bindra, B. Fairclough, and A. Westcombe. 1993. Culture and body image: Body perception and weight concern in young Asian and Caucasian British women. *Journal of Community and Applied Social Psychology* 3:173–181.

Wardle, J., S. Carnell, C. M. A. Haworth, and R. Plomin. 2008. Evidence for a strong genetic influence on childhood adiposity despite the force of the obesogenic environment. *American Journal of Clinical Nutrition* 87(2): 398–404.

Waxler, N. 1998. Learning to be a leper: A case study in the social construction of illness. In *Understanding and Applying Medical Anthropology*, ed. P. Brown, 147–157. Toronto: Mayfield.

Weber, L., and E. Fore. 2007. Race, ethnicity, and health: An intersectional approach. In *Handbook of the Sociology of Racial and Ethnic Relations*, ed. J. Feagin and H. Vera, 191–218. New York: Springer.

Weiss, E. C., D. A. Galuska, K. L. Kettel, C. Gillespie, and M. K. Serdula. 2007. Weight regain in U.S. adults who experienced substantial weight loss, 1999–2002. *American Journal of Preventive Medicine* 33(1): 34–40.

Weller, S. C. 2007. Cultural consensus theory: Applications and frequently asked questions. *Field Methods* 19(4): 339–368.

Wellman, B. 1979. The community question: The intimate networks of East Yorkers. *American Journal of Sociology* 84:1201–1231.

Wells, J.C.K. 2006. The evolution of human fatness and susceptibility to obesity: An ethological approach. *Biological Reviews* 81:183–205.

———. 2007. The thrifty phenotype as an adaptive maternal effect. *Biological Reviews* 82(1): 143–172.

Whitacre, T. P., P. Tsai, and J. Mulligan. 2009. *The Public Health Effects of Food Deserts*. Washington, D.C.: National Academies Press.

White, M. 2007. Food access and obesity. *Obesity Reviews* 8:99–107.

WHO [World Health Organization]. 1995. *Physical Status: The Use and Interpretation of Anthropometry*. WHO Technical Report Series. Geneva: World Health Organization.

———. 1998. *Obesity: Preventing and Managing the Global Epidemic: Report of a WHO Consultation on Obesity*. Geneva: World Health Organization.

———. 2004. Appropriate body-mass index for Asian populations and its implications for policy and intervention strategies. *Lancet* 363:157–163.

———. 2010. World Health Organization global database on BMI. *http://apps.who.int/bmi/index.jsp*. Accessed March 2010.

Wildman, R. P., P. Muntner, K. Reynolds, A. P. McGinn, S. Rajpathak, J. Wylie-Rosett, and M. R. Sowers. 2008. The obese without cardiometabolic risk factor clustering and the normal weight with cardiometabolic risk factor clustering: Prevalence and correlates of 2 phenotypes among the U.S. population (NHANES 1999–2004). *Archives of Internal Medicine* 168(15): 1617–1624.

Wilkes, C. 1856. *Narrative of the United States Exploring Expedition during the Years 1838*, 1939, 1840, 1841, 1842. Vol. 2. Philadelphia: Lea and Blanchard.

Wilkinson, J. Y., D. I. Ben-Tovim, and M. K. Walker. 1994. An insight into the personal and cultural significance of weight and shape in large Samoan women. *International Journal of Obesity* 18:602–606.

Williamson, D. A., L. G. Womble, N. L. Zucker, D. L. Reas, M. A. White, D. C. Blouin, and F. Greenway. 2000. Body image assessment for obesity (BIA-O): Development of a new procedure. *International Journal of Obesity and Related Metabolic Disorders* 24(10): 1326–1332.

Wilson, D. K. 2009. New perspectives on health disparities and obesity interventions in youth. *Journal of Pediatric Psychology* 34(3): 231–244.

Wolf, A. M. 1998. What is the economic case for treating obesity? *Obesity Research* 6(1): 2S–7S.

Wolf, A. M., and G. A. Colditz. 1998. Current estimates of the economic cost of obesity in the United States. *Obesity Research* 6(2): 97–106.

Worldwatch Institute. 2000. *State of the World 2000: A Worldwatch Institute Report on Progress toward Sustainable Society*. New York: W. W. Norton

Worthman, C. M. 1994. Developmental microniche: A concept for modeling relationships of biology, behavior, and culture in development. *American Journal of Physical Anthropology* 37(S18): 210.

———. 1996. Biosocial determinants of sex ratios: Survivorship, selection, and socialization in the early environment. In *Long Term Consequences of Early Environment: Growth, Development, and the Lifespan Developmental Perspective*, ed. C.J.K. Henry and S. J. Ulijaszek, 44–68. Cambridge: Cambridge University Press.

Worthman, C. M., C. L. Jenkins, J. F. Stallings, and D. Lai. 1993. Attenuation of nursing-related ovarian suppression and high fertility in well-nourished, intensively breast-feeding Amele women of Lowland Papua New Guinea. *Journal of Biosocial Science* 25:425–443.

Worthman, C. M., and B. Kohrt. 2005. Receding horizons of health: Biocultural approaches to public health paradoxes. *Social Science and Medicine* 61(4, 8): 861–878.

Wrigley, N., D. Warm, and B. Margetts. 2003. Deprivation, diet, and food-retail access: Findings from the Leeds 'food deserts' study. *Environment and Planning* A35:151–188.

Wrigley, N., D. Warm, B. Margetts, and A. Whelan. 2002. Assessing the impact of improved retail access on diet in a 'food desert.' *Urban Studies* 39:2061–2082.

Wutich, A., and C. McCarty. 2008. Social networks and infant feeding in Oaxaca, Mexico. *Maternal and Child Nutrition* 4:121–135.

Yu, D. W., and G. H. Shepard. 1998. Is beauty in the eye of the beholder? *Nature* 396:321–322.

Zdrodowski, D. 1996. Eating out: The experience of eating in public for the overweight woman. *Women's Studies International Forum* 19(60): 655–664.

Zhiqin, L., Y. Zhou, C. Carter-Su, M. G. Myers Jr., and L. Rui. 2007. SH2B1 enhances leptin signaling by both Janus Kinase 2 Tyr813-dependent and -independent mechanisms. *Molecular Endocrinology* 21(9): 2270–2281.

Zimmet, P., S. Faaiuso, J. Ainuu, S. Whitehouse, B. Milne, and W. DeBoer. 1981. The prevalence of diabetes in the rural and urban Polynesian population of Western Samoa. *Diabetes* 30:45–51.

INDEX

Page numbers in *italics* refer to figures and tables.

ABOUT THE AUTHOR

A New Zealander by birth, Alexandra Brewis Slade has lived and done research globally, including Mexico, the Pacific Islands, and the southern United States. She currently lives with her family in sunny Tempe, Arizona, where she holds positions as professor of medical anthropology, director of the Center for Global Health, and executive director of the School of Human Evolution and Social Change at Arizona State University. In addition to managing field-research projects in Arizona and elsewhere, she keeps busy teaching anthropology and managing a suite of study abroad programs for undergraduates in such places as China, Fiji, and London. Alex holds MA and PhD degrees in anthropology from the University of Auckland and University of Arizona respectively, and did postdoctoral study in demography at Brown University.